YOGA

An Hachette UK Company
www.hachette.co.uk

First published in Great Britain in 2021 by
Godsfield, an imprint of
Octopus Publishing Group Ltd
Carmelite House
50 Victoria Embankment
London EC4Y 0DZ
www.octopusbooks.co.uk
www.octopusbooksusa.com

Distributed in the US by
Hachette Book Group
1290 Avenue of the Americas
4th and 5th Floors
New York, NY 10104

Distributed in Canada by
Canadian Manda Group
664 Annette St.
Toronto, Ontario, Canada M6S 2C8

ISBN 978-1-84181-493-3

A CIP catalogue record for this book is available
from the British Library.

Printed and bound in China

10 9 8 7 6 5 4 3 2 1

All reasonable care has been taken in the
preparation of this book but the information
it contains is not intended to take the place
treatment by a qualified medical practitioner.

Before making any changes in your health
regime, always consult a doctor. While
all the therapies detailed in this book are
completely safe if done correctly, you must
seek professional advice if you are in any doubt
about any medical condition. Any application
of the ideas and information contained in this
book is at the reader's sole discretion and risk.

Publishing Director: Stephanie Jackson
Art Director: Yasia Williams-Leedham
Senior Production Controller: Emily Noto

Project Editor: Clare Churly
Copy-editor: Mandy Greenfield
Designer: Leonardo Collina
Illustrator: Emilia Franchini

YOGA

THE GUIDE TO POSES, PRACTICES AND MORE

Lucy Lucas

Contents

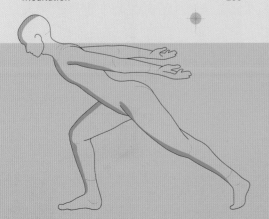

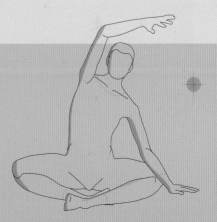

Preface

It was a sandwich board on my local shopping street that drew my attention:
a beginners' yoga course. Fifteen months had passed since my back surgery
and I wasn't in any pain, but I had heard that yoga was good for backs, and for
busy lives in general, so together with a friend, I signed up. Several weeks of
breathing, which I hated at first, gentle movement and self-inquiry later, I was
a convert. In that quiet, softly lit space I felt as if I had come home.

Yoga is all about coming home: to ourselves. We arrive in the world unbroken, and
yet life conditions us to feel otherwise, leaving us disconnected and slightly lost.
This was me 11 years ago when I first stepped onto the yoga path, and over time
its practices and worldview, or philosophy, have brought me much closer to who
I truly am, who I always was – peeling back the hardened layers that I adopted as
self-protection.

I have practised all kinds of physical yoga, from Ashtanga to restorative yoga, from
Iyengar to mindful movement. I have experienced a wide range of breathing and
meditation techniques, and have read and discussed so much about how yogis
– yoga experts – see the world. When I first learned to teach, it was in a precise,
alignment-based style that ultimately didn't work for my body. I thought for a long
time there was something wrong with me, rather than questioning the practices
themselves. When I learned that much of our modern postural yoga was designed
in a specific milieu for a specific population, I understood that it wasn't my body at
fault, and that maybe we could change the way we move to better suit 21st-century
bodies and lifestyles.

Even a short review of yoga's history, such as is given in this book (see pages
16–22), will hopefully show how yoga has changed and adapted over time.
Yogis have long been taking existing worldviews and practices and exploring and
experimenting with them, bringing new methods and ways of thinking, adapting
and improvising, in order to arrive at an approach that works in a specific era.
We are now in a place where everything is uncertain and existing boundaries are
being rewritten. In this era we need a practice that is adaptable to change, but one
that gives us the grounding and centring we require, in order to face the constant
upheavals that we have to confront.

This book provides a short overview of the different types of yoga, its history and philosophy. We then look at how yoga works physically in the body: not just the poses, but also how breathwork and meditation impact on our nervous system. Poses, sequences and other practices are included to help cultivate awareness and a sense of exploration. Curiosity about how the body–mind responds to certain practices – what works and what doesn't – has always been part of the yogic path, and it is this spirit of self-inquiry that I hope fills this book, and your ongoing yoga practice.

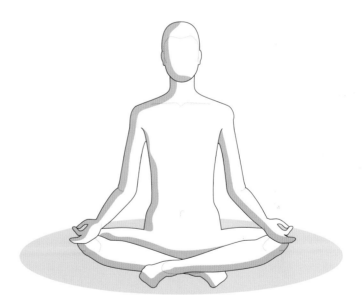

1
WHAT IS
YOGA?

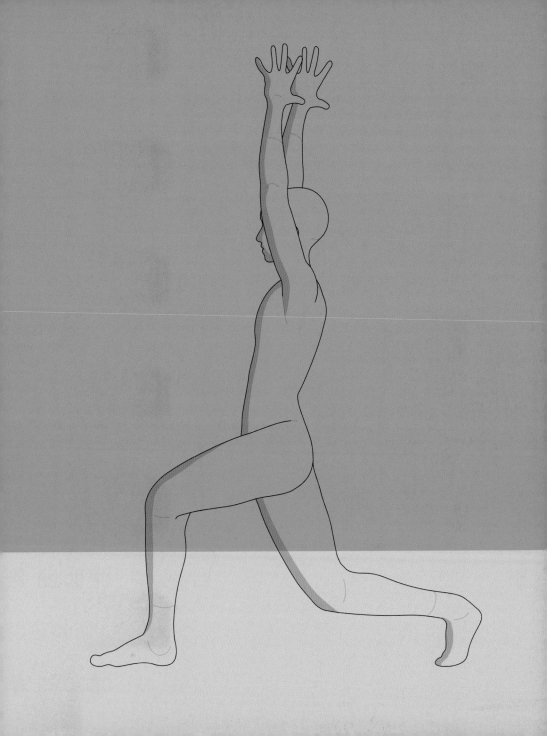

What is Yoga?

There are thought to be around 300 million yoga practitioners worldwide, with an estimated $80 billion spent on yoga each year. Despite its global takeover, yoga is often conflated with a physical exercise regime or with feeling less stressed. Focus in the West is on the practices of yoga: the *asanas* or postures, breathing, relaxation and so on. If we ask ourselves what the purpose of these practices is, then our goals tend to be quite narrow and short-term: stress reduction, help for our sore backs and becoming more flexible.

Yet something else also emerges, especially among longer-term practitioners. In my own experience, yoga helped me realize that the life I was living was profoundly not right for me, and gave me the courage to change it. Many other people have switched jobs, moved countries, left unhelpful relationships, begun new relationships, started businesses and made numerous other major changes. What is it about moving our bodies, breathing and being still in particular ways that takes us from feeling a bit better, when we leave the studio, to making huge life-changing decisions?

To answer that question, we need to look at why people traditionally practised yoga (the goal) and what they were practising in order to get there (the practices). The goals and practices of yoga have stayed the same over time, and yet they have always shifted, depending on the environment at a particular time. More than 2,000 years ago the Sramanas (see page 16) were predominantly interested in mind-control practices, to liberate them from the endless cycle of birth and rebirth. Today, yoga practitioners are more interested in ways they can relax and reconnect with themselves as an antidote to everyday stress. Both are ways of finding freedom from types of suffering, and both involve practices that are ancient and modern.

The goal, or outcome, of yoga is said to be liberation (*moksa*) from suffering. In the time of the Sramanas, suffering was thought to be the cycle of birth and rebirth. Today, suffering is the back ache of sedentary or physical jobs; lack of mobility; lack of respite from the constant stimulation and demands on our time; our ancient neurological wiring struggling to cope in the 21st century; anxiety and worry about ourselves, our kids and the planet. Suffering is the trauma and conditioning held in the body, which affects our daily lives. It is the stories and beliefs that limit our potential. Most of us can recognize some of that suffering – it's universal.

The yogis developed complex philosophical systems to describe reality, the universe and our relationship and role within it, and these philosophies are still relevant today. A lot of our pain is caused by believing certain things about ourselves, others and the world, without ever fully inquiring into their actual truth. We are often attached to certain things, or dislike others, without fully asking why, or whether we can be free from them. Yoga asks us to come into our actual experience in the moment and really be there, in all its facets, so that we can start to see what is real for us and what might be conditioned in us.

Over time, yoga has developed a number of methods to help free us from this suffering. The body plays a crucial role in this, as we use yogic practices to manage energy in the body, which affects our emotional and mental states. Yoga postures (*asanas*) provide a means of grounding, connecting, embodiment (feeling more deeply connected with our bodies) and a way of changing our state. Meditation and mind management can help us create a new relationship with our thoughts and emotions. We can manage energy in the body through *pranayama* breathwork (see page 252), visualization and mantras (a group of words or syllables). And we can take the practice off the mat, by reviewing and applying yoga philosophies for approaching daily life.

Yoga and Religion

Yoga is an ancient Indian tradition, and it has both influenced some religions and been part of others over the course of its history. Yoga itself is not a religion, but started as a break-away movement of renunciant men called Sramanas, around 500 BCE. One of these men, Gautama Buddha, took early yogic practices from this movement (see page 16), added mindfulness (paying attention in the present moment) and set out across India to spread the word of Buddhism. The Sramana movement also gave rise to Jainism, another of India's great religions.

In the early medieval period the religion of Saivism was the crucible in which Tantric yoga (see page 13) flourished, not only in terms of practice, but also in terms of the philosophical thinking that underpinned it. Tantric yoga influenced many other traditions across India and Asia. When Europeans arrived in India in the late-medieval period, they were confronted by a myriad of different religions and beliefs, and the British coined the term "Hindustan", meaning east of the Indus River. All religions that were not Islam, Buddhism or Jainism started to come under the term "Hinduism", including Saivism, Vaishnavism and more Brahminical traditions – those considered to have the highest social status. A religion is considered to be Hindu if it can trace its origin back to the Vedas, the most ancient of Indian scriptures (see page 16). There has been an effort in recent years to reclaim yoga as being particularly Hindu, even though yoga pre-dates the cultural idea of Hinduism in either religious or cultural terms by more than 1,000 years.

Today this cross-fertilization between yoga practices and religion is played out in different ways. For some people, yoga is closely related to religious practice; for others, there is a considerable non-religious devotional element. Bhakti yoga (see below) is a spiritual practice that is co-created by the practitioner and the tradition. Typically this includes acknowledging the divine in yourself and finding greater connection to self, to others, to the community and to the planet. Mindfulness, Zen practices and Buddhist Tantra are all examples of the cross-fertilization of yoga and Buddhism.

There is no need to adopt a particular religious or cultural identity to practise yoga unless you feel this is important for you, or unless it is a part of your heritage that you wish to connect to. All the practices of yoga can be explored regardless of religious background.

Different Types of Yoga

There are many different forms of yoga, both in terms of outcome and practice. Below are some of the types that you may hear referenced, and the era from which they come.

From the Pre-Modern Era

The first four of these types of yoga are specifically mentioned in the Bhagavad Gita scripture.

- **Karma yoga**: the yoga of action without attachment to the result.
- **Bhakti yoga**: the yoga of devotion (to the divine).
- **Jnana yoga**: the yoga of wisdom and knowledge, of your true nature, of understanding the nature of reality.
- **Abhyasa yoga**: the yoga of continued practice.
- **Classical yoga**: the yoga of Patanjali, the compiler of the *Yoga Sutras* (see page 16): focus on meditation and concentration.

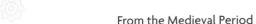

From the Medieval Period

- **Tantric yoga**: various spiritual traditions such as Saivism, using embodiment techniques – for instance, visualization, meditation and the use of deities – to cultivate awareness of your true nature.
- **Hatha yoga**: the yoga of movement, using the body and the breath to manage *prana*, or energy, to experience altered states.
- **Raja yoga**: the royal yoga, specifically meaning the yoga of meditation.

Modern Yoga

The first five of these types of modern yoga were defined by yoga historian Elizabeth De Michelis.

- **Psychosomatic yoga**: the interconnectedness of the physical, emotional and mental in our experience, as popularized by the yoga of Swami Vivekananda (1863–1902); it is very influential across all modern yoga.
- **Hindu/Nationalist yoga**: from the late 19th century through to Indian independence, this focused on the Indian – and especially Hindu – roots of yoga; now undergoing a strong revival.
- **Denominational yoga**: focuses more explicitly on doctrine and the practice of devotion and service toward a manifestation of the divine, which is called *bhakti*.
- **Meditational yoga**: focuses on a specific set of meditations rather than on postural practices; it is more likely to have an explicit ideological content and may overlap with denominational yoga – for example, the Transcendental Meditation of Maharishi Mahesh Yogi.
- **Postural yoga**: puts an emphasis on *asanas*, or poses, and movement, and may or may not have a doctrinal underpinning – for instance, Iyengar yoga or Vinyasa yoga (see page 14).
- **Post-lineage yoga**: represents the emergence of postural, *bhakti* and meditation yoga practices outside traditional lineages and denominations, as defined by Theodora Wildcroft, a researcher of contemporary yoga.

Postural Yoga

Here are the eight main types of postural yoga that you might hear of, or see advertised at studios.

Ashtanga Yoga

Ashtanga yoga is a set series of poses devised by K Pattabhi Jois, a student of T Krishnamacharya (see pages 18–19) in Mysore, India. In a teacher-led Ashtanga class, students follow the instructor through the defined sequence and the class completes them together. In a Mysore-style class, students follow the series by themselves and the teacher will help individual students where necessary, allowing them to progress at their own speed, with their own breath. Teachers may also perform adjustments on students to help them into a deeper version of the pose. If you don't want to be touched or adjusted, you should inform the teacher at the start of the class.

Vinyasa Yoga

This is probably one of the most available forms of modern postural yoga today in the West. Derived from the Ashtanga system of moving from pose to pose with the breath, Vinyasa yoga doesn't follow a standard sequence, thereby allowing teachers greater freedom and creativity with their classes. Sequences are arranged around Sun Salutations, with variations added to the core poses; or they may include a series of postures interspersed with a shortened Sun Salutation in the middle. The speed of the sequence will depend on the type and level of the class, and on the teacher. Similar styles include flow, dynamic, power, rocket, Baptiste, Anusara and Jivamukti yoga.

Hatha Yoga

Hatha classes tend to be denoted as slower, less dynamic, with more focus on seated *pranayama* and meditation exercises. These classes can be just as challenging as the more dynamic ones, because holding poses with stability and muscle engagement is not easy. Similar classes might be called classical or traditional yoga, or by a specific name such as Sivananda yoga.

Iyengar Yoga

B K S Iyengar was another student of Krishnamacharya in Mysore. Iyengar is a form of Hatha yoga, with a focus on alignment, control and precision. Students start with more simple poses and progress to more complex ones over time. Iyengar yoga makes extensive use of props and equipment to assist students in exploring the poses. For a more dynamic practice, Anusara yoga is based on similar, but less precise, principles and is more of a Vinyasa flow-style.

Restorative Yoga

Restorative yoga is designed for relaxation and rest. Poses are usually floor-based, mainly involve lying down and use lots of props to ensure the body is fully supported. Poses can be held for upward of five to ten minutes, and the teacher will often guide meditations or gentle breathing exercises, or may even read poems during this time.

Yin Yoga

Yin yoga draws on Traditional Chinese Medicine (TCM) as well as yoga. The intention behind the practice is to allow muscles to relax, then to add stress to other tissues: ligaments, tendons, fascia and joints. Through these poses the TCM meridians, or energy pathways, can be affected. Poses are mainly floor-based, either lying or seated, and props may be used. Poses are held from two to five minutes, and sometimes longer. Yin yoga works well with a mindfulness practice, as it specifically cultivates the attitude of non-striving and the practice of "letting be".

Hot Yoga

Hot yoga is practised in a heated room with temperatures of 30–37°C (86–98.6°F). Any style of yoga can be done in the heat, from Vinyasa to Hatha, but hot yoga is perhaps most famously known through Bikram yoga – a set sequence of poses practised in the heat, as popularized by Bikram Choudhury.

Post-Lineage Yoga

Almost all modern postural yoga can be traced back to a few main lineages, such as Ashtanga or Iyengar yoga. Dedication and devotion to a teacher and lineage have often created an adherence to rules and protocols, not all of which are helpful. As the result of an increase in injuries, and the abuse of power by some gurus, there is now a movement toward a yoga that is not beholden to any one style. This post-lineage yoga incorporates different styles of movement, such as Feldenkrais and Pilates, and includes a variety of other practices, from meditation to breathwork and spiritual and devotional themes, not all of which are necessarily Indian.

The History of Yoga

The word "yoga" has many meanings, depending on the context in which it is used. It is both goal and practice; a verb meaning "to yoke" or join together; and can also mean magic or a business transaction. One of the earliest mentions of yoga belongs to the Vedic period – a Brahminical society that existed in India c.5000–1000 BCE. The Vedas are a set of divinely inspired texts that underpin Hinduism. In the Atharva Veda, yoga is used in the context of yoking animals.

Around 500 BCE civilization in this area started to change: from a ritualistic society to one with more critical thinking, a greater emphasis on the individual and a focus on the ideas of liberation and awakening. This context gave rise to the Sramana movement, an underground group of men who gave up everyday life for spiritual inquiry and practice. This included breath control (*pranayama*), meditation and various austerities (*tapas*) designed to discipline or "yoke" the mind to find altered states of consciousness. One of the most famous Sramanas is Gautama Buddha, whose practices and mindfulness innovation led to the religion of Buddhism.

The Bhagavad Gita is part of the Mahabarata epic and a canonical text of Brahmanism. This text is one of many Upanishads, written around 800–200 BCE, and is seen as a reconciliation between worldly life and renunciation. We see a conversation between the god Krishna and the soldier Arjuna at a moment when a key battle is about to take place. Krishna is placed as the supreme yogi, as he guides Arjuna on whether or not he should fight his kinsmen. Key concepts such as *karmayoga* (yoga of action) and *bhaktiyoga* (yoga of devotion) are explained by Krishna. In the use of a god, Krishna, and a young king, Arjuna, social norms and Brahmanical traditions are reinforced.

The *Yoga Sutras* of Patanjali are a short text of 196 *sutras*, or concise statements and associated commentary, about yogic states and practices to achieve them, including the well-known Eight-Limbed Path, or Ashtanga yoga. The *Yoga Sutras* are mainly about meditation and were compiled for renunciant men. They list *samadhi* as the final step on the path to the goal of yoga – a deep trance state said to eradicate *samskaras*, or energy knots, in the mind and body, which influence current thoughts and behaviours.

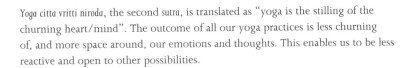

Yoga citta vritti niroda, the second *sutra*, is translated as "yoga is the stilling of the churning heart/mind". The outcome of all our yoga practices is less churning of, and more space around, our emotions and thoughts. This enables us to be less reactive and open to other possibilities.

Around 500 CE we see the rise of the spiritual tradition called Tantra across the north-western part of India, against a backdrop of warring kingdoms and uncertainty. Although it is not a religion itself, Tantra arose from Saivism, and aspects of it passed into other religions, such as Buddhism, and spread to southern India and Indonesia. Tantra included rituals, a specific worldview and new ways of practising yoga. The aim was liberation (*moksa*) through union with the deity, which Saivism is organized around. Liberation was seen as possible within this life, but it was also possible to have material goals as well.

Initiation (*diksa*) into the tradition by a guru was critical, but this was open to anyone, including women, householders and lower castes. Tantra also developed a sophisticated model of the subtle body through which *prana* can be directed. Also featured was the repetition of mantras, whose sounds are said to be manifestations of the deities. Many aspects of Tantric yoga are part of modern yoga, such as the *chakra* system (see page 248).

Following the Muslim invasion of northern India in c.1200 CE, the lack of funding of Tantric institutions, and the decline in the number of householders practising it, meant that renunciants again became the main holders of yogic traditions.

One meaning of *hatha* is force, and Hatha yoga became known for its austere physical practices. The goals were again liberation (*moksa*) and powers (*siddhis*); these were to be achieved by raising an energy called Kundalini: the latent consciousness or goddess power that is coiled at the base of the spine. Practices are designed so that Kundalini rise ups the spine to achieve union with the god Shiva, and thus liberation. Hatha yoga was also said to be important for *Rajayoga* or *Samadhi* – meditative consciousness.

The main text of Hatha yoga is the *Hathapradipika* of *c*.1450, which included postures (*asanas*), *pranayama* and cleansing practices (*satkarma*). The Hatha yoga period was also known for the interest in the physical benefits of practice, such as preventing old age. The *Hathapradipika* includes 15 *asanas*, including the Bow (Dhanurasana) and a seated twist (Matsyendrasana). *Asana* is said to lead to steadiness, health and suppleness. A later text, the *Hathabhyasapaddhati* of the 1700s, has a section on *asana* that contains six groups of poses arranged into specific sequences. It is thought likely that T Krishnamacharya (see below), one of the most influential teachers of modern postural yoga, knew of this book.

The Hatha yoga period is when yoga became much more physical, with a focus on improving health and living to an old age. It is these two themes that have been consistent throughout the rest of yoga's history, into the 19th and 20th centuries and up to the present day.

In the late 19th century there was an explosion of interest in the practice of health and fitness, often expressed in terms of the individual's duty to the nation. The British enthusiasm for gymnastics, wrestling and bodybuilding was matched by that of Indians, and occurred at the start of a concerted fight-back against the colonial power. The idea of the "strong Indian" was born from Indians' desire to counteract part of a colonial stereotype that had been internalized to justify British supremacy. This idea – that Indian men were effeminate and weak – made wrestling and bodybuilding very popular among Indians, and many aspects of these movements were incorporated into yoga *asana* sequences in later decades.

It was also during this time that yoga made a transition from being a practice for renunciants into one for householders, and a key factor was the focus on its health and therapeutic benefits. Institutes such as Shri Yogendra's Yoga Institute and the Vivekananda Yoga Kendra were places where this mix of health, therapeutics and a wider democratization of yoga was spread.

Indians wanted to disseminate the teachings of yoga – and their traditions – more widely. This cross-cultural influence grew with visits to the West from important yoga gurus from various traditions. In 1893 Swami Vivekananda travelled to Chicago to attend and speak at the World Parliament of Religions, an interfaith conference, followed by a US and European speaking tour, and published his book *Raja Yoga* in 1896.

The Maharaja Krishnaraja Wadiyar IV asked T Krishnamacharya to start a yoga school in the 1920s–1930s at the Mysore Palace to popularize a form of physical culture rooted in India's traditions. His students were typically Indian adolescent men, and the yoga *asanas* and sequences developed there (many of which are still practised) were developed for them and their bodies – a context that is sometimes overlooked when Westerners are practising yoga today.

Four pupils of Krishnamacharya went on to have a considerable impact on the development of yoga in the West. K Pattabhi Jois developed a strong, athletic form called Ashtanga yoga (see page 14). B K S Iyengar created his self-named precise form of yoga (see page 14) using lots of props; many of the *asana* names and alignment instructions come from his teaching. Indra Devi worked in Hollywood during the late 1940s and early 1950s, teaching many famous stars. And Krishnamacharya's son, T K V Desikachar, developed a more personalized yoga called Viniyoga, which has many followers.

After the Second World War yoga continued its influence in the West as part of the 1960s counterculture, and a proliferation of yoga schools was established, such as the Sivananda ashrams and yoga adult-education classes. Popular music stars promoted yoga in the 1990s, with Sting and Madonna making famous the rigorous Ashtanga yoga. Yoga in the 21st century is now ubiquitous and is well known for its health benefits.

What becomes clear, when we review the tangled knots of yoga's history, is its constant evolution: a renewal of practices and goals situated in the environment of the time. Modern postural yoga, for example, is a mix of Hatha yoga postures, Tantric *prana* techniques, Western gymnastics and Buddhist mindfulness. Today yoga is largely about health and wellbeing, a trend that, although it is several hundred years old, is required to combat our often sedentary and stress-filled lives. Amid this continual change, however, we must remember the traditions that evolved to give us our modern practices, and must honour the culture and history that created them.

YOGA HISTORY TIMELINE

Dates	Main types of yoga	Yoga events	Yoga texts	Indian and world events
1500–1000 BCE			c.1700–1000 BCE: Rig Veda mentions the long-haired one. c.1000 BCE: Atharva Veda mentions yoga in the context of yoking.	Vedic period: Ritualistic society based on sacrifices to the gods.
1000–0 BCE	Sramana movement: The start of yoga.	c.600 BCE: Jainism founded. c.480–400 BCE: The Buddha studies with the Sramanas and travels to spread his teachings.	c.800–500 BCE: The Upanishads. c.400–200 BCE: The Mahabharata, including the Bhagavad Gita.	Collective rise of critical thinking, with more focus on the individual; increased migration, urbanization and multiculturalism.
0–700 CE	Classical	Influence of Sankhya and Vedanta philosophy.	325–425 CE: The Yoga Sutras of Patanjali. 350 CE: Sankhya Karika (Isvara Krishna). 700 CE: Brahma Sutras (Shankara).	Birth of Christ. 300–500 CE: Gupta Empire.
700–1200	Tantric	c.600–1200: Tantric yoga institutionalized. Spread of Tantra to Indonesia.	c.1000: Vijnana Bhairava Tantra; The Recognition Sutras (Ksemaraja); and Tantraloka (Abhinavagupta).	900: Beginning of Muslim invasions to northern India. Flourishing of kingdoms in Kashmir and southern India.

Dates	Main types of yoga	Yoga events	Yoga texts	Indian and world events
1200–1800	Hatha	Yoga goes underground. 1500: Nath and other movements gain ground; wandering holy men.	c.1100–1300: *Goraksasataka* (Gorakhnath) and *Dattatrayogasastra* (Dattatreya). c.1450: *Hathapradipika* (Swatmarama).	1300s: Culmination of Muslim invasions. 1400s: First main contact of Europeans in India. 1757–1858: Rule of India by the British East India Company.
1800s	19th-century revival	1893: Swami Vivekananda visits USA and Europe. Increased focus on the health and wellbeing benefits of yoga in India.	1893: *Raja Yoga* (Vivekananda).	1858: British colonial rule of India – the Raj.
1920s–1950s	Mysore Revival	1920s–1930s: T Krishnamacharya teaches K P Jois, B Y S Iyengar, T K V Desikachar and Indra Devi. 1936: Divine Life Society (Vedanta) founded. 1940s/1950s: Indra Devi teaches Hollywood stars.	1953: *Forever Young, Forever Healthy: Simplified Yoga for Modern Living* (Indra Devi).	1919: Amritsar Massacre. 1939–1945: Second World War. 1947: Indian independence.

Dates	Main types of yoga	Yoga events	Yoga texts	Indian and world events
1960s–1990s	Modern postural yoga	1960s: Bihar and Sivananda schools of yoga founded. 1964: B K S Iyengar visits Europe for the first time. 1968: The Beatles visit Rishikesh ashram in India. 1969: Satchidananda Saraswati speaks at Woodstock. 1990s: Ashtanga popularized by Sting and Madonna.	1966: *Light on Yoga* (B K S Iyengar).	1960s–1970s: Countercultural movement. 1980s: Development of Mindfulness-Based Stress Reduction programme by Jon Kabat-Zinn.
2000s	Posti-lineage yoga	Growth and proliferation of yoga studios, teachers and styles. 2018: Revelation of sexual assaults by gurus.	2010: *Yoga Body* (Mark Singleton).	Increased societal focus on wellbeing and stress reduction.

Yoga Philosophy

Philosophy means a worldview, *darshana* in Sanskrit – a way of understanding how our world is constructed, and how we relate to it. Worldviews helps us to contextualize our practice and think about why we are here in the first place.

Due to its rich history, India has had many philosophies, but one of the most influential is Sankyha. The *Sankhya Karika* by Isvara Krishna is thought to have originated in the 4th century CE, roughly at the same time as Patanjali's *Yoga Sutras*. Sankyha establishes a fundamental duality in the universe between the masculine *purusha* and the feminine *prakrti*. *Purusha* is pure consciousness: no form, no shape, a witness; *prakrti* is everything else in the material world. When *purusha* and *prakrti* get close, the universe manifests, as it needs both pure energy (consciousness) and matter to come into being.

The manifested universe is seen as comprising 25 elements, known as *tattvas*, and these have certain qualities known as *gunas*. These qualities are seen in everything: from our personalities, to the nervous system, the food we eat, the activities we do. See pages 276–278 for a broader explanation of how we experience the *gunas* effect. In Sankhya the practitioner is attempting to separate *purusha* from *prakrti*, to overcome the manifest (the material world) and unite with pure consciousness.

Another key philosophy is Vedanta, of which there are several schools of thought, the most popular being Advaita Vedanta. The main teachings come from the *Brahma Sutras* by Shankara around 700 CE and are influenced by Sankyha, which pre-dates it. Advaita Vedanta is non-dual, and in this "everything is one" perspective we have an individual self (Atman) and a pure consciousness (Brahman). Atman is the same as Brahman – we are all part of one big field of energy. Any identification with the material universe, any ideas of being separate from consciousness or from others, is considered to be simply an illusion. All is one.

Sankyha forms the key philosophical backbone to Patanjali's *Yoga Sutras*, and many yoga practices are based on this dualism. However, Vedanta is also very pervasive in modern yoga, due to Swami Vivekananda, who followed his initial visit to the West in the 1890s by setting up Vedanta Societies throughout the USA and beyond. Vedanta was also the school of thought behind Sivananda and his disciples, and the yoga schools that followed.

This simple dichotomy is not reflected in the range of Indian thought, however. The Bhagavad Gita is a famous example of a very common view in India – that of *bhedabheda*, which posits that the divine is in everything, but is not the whole of everything. Some schools of Tantra go one step further than even the whole dual vs non-dual debate, and state that all of these possibilities exist, but they are subsumed by a higher non-duality that takes precedence.

Awareness

The relationship with ourselves and the universe depends on how we perceive our experience of reality. How we perceive, how we feel and how we know anything at all are parts of being aware. Yoga practice is primarily about cultivating awareness: the poses and meditation are merely tools to help us practise this, in terms of where we are in space on the floor, how we feel and what effect the practice has on us. Awareness occurs through our senses, our nervous system, internal embodiment and mind, and creates that real sense of "knowing". Some of this knowing will derive from our conditioning: we observe a table, but we only know it as a table due to our experience.

Worldview also influences awareness in the relationship between the perceiver and perceived. In Sankyha the separation of *purusha* and *prakrti* can be experienced through the observation of *prakrti*/matter rather than identifying with it. In our modern yoga practice, a simple exercise might be to observe the breath or a candle flame, therefore experiencing what it is to be an observer. Here I am, watching my breath, where "I" is *purusha*, or awareness, and the breath is *prakrti* or material existence. Our experience of awareness is thought of as one of withdrawal and separation.

Tantrics argued that it was difficult to draw a line between perceiver and perceived. For example, if we watch the breath in meditation, there is an effect on us, the watcher: we often become calmer and more centred, even after a short period. We always bring our previous experiences, stories, beliefs and conditioning to every moment and every object that we perceive. In the Tantric model, this relationship between awareness and object can only happen if they are the same thing.

Does anything even exist outside of our awareness? There is the subtle acknowledgement that all existence is part of one same field of awareness. It is sometimes described as the silence behind sounds: sound would not exist without silence to hold it. Likewise, the idea of a fish wondering what all this water is. It is such an integral part of his experience that he never questions it.

Unclear Seeing

If cultivation of awareness lies at the heart of the yoga journey, what are the things along the path that prevent us from clear seeing? In Sankhya there are the five "afflictions" (*kleshas*), which are conditioned beliefs and behaviours that keep us stuck in the dark. These afflictions are ignorance (*avidya*) of our true nature; small self (*asmita*); attraction (*raga*); aversion (*dvesha*) and clinging (*abhinivesha*): clinging to life and avoiding death in an attempt to avoid the vast, impermanent state of what life really is.

We live in a world in which we are overly identified with surface reality: our physical bodies; our material possessions; our thoughts and our religious and political beliefs. This ignorance of our wider consciousness and connection is seen as the cause of suffering. It obscures reality and confuses us as to who we are and why we are here. Ignorance can leave us feeling disconnected, estranged and empty: we try to fill the hole with more possessions, another relationship, and so on. Liberation comes from bringing awareness to this condition and seeing that there is more to life than we may currently perceive.

In medieval Tantric yoga the three impurities (*malas*), or perceptions, provide a similar concept. The Impurity of Individuality is the unconscious belief that there is something wrong with us, or something missing, and is considered the primary cause of suffering. The Impurity of Differentiation means that we only ever see the differences between us and others, and not the similarities. It helps to remember that we are all imperfect people living imperfect lives – this is our common humanity. The Impurity of Action (karma), says that if we see ourselves as separate and limited, this necessarily drives our desire to acquire more and give ourselves an advantage over others. This illusion is linked to the *kleshas* of aversion and attraction (see above): the need for something outside ourselves to find peace or feel fulfilled.

The solution is to address the root of the action: the feeling of lack, or fear, that drives the clinging and pushing away. The way out of separation is to reflect upon our common humanity, and the path from ignorance is one of awakening: to understand that anything else is suffering too, but that more exists beyond.

Understanding Conditioning

We are all conditioned, because we arrive unformed and then are moulded into adult humans. Conditioning comes from family, school, society and culture, religion and other environmental events, and is expressed in our anatomy, physiology, beliefs, appearance, behaviour, thoughts and emotions. Conditioning is also passed down the generations through society and culture, family dynamics, parenting styles and common beliefs. The yogic practice starts with noticing the story and watching the impact of conditioning upon you.

The energy of this conditioning is believed, in the yogic system, to affect not only our physical structure but also to penetrate the energy of the subtle body (see page 246). Stressful thoughts, trauma, and every event and experience are collated in the physical and energy bodies. These contractions create energy knots (*samskaras*), which we are often unconscious of until we do deep, energetic body work. Unwinding *samskaras* can be painful, especially when it involves questioning long-held beliefs and when those beliefs are shared with others.

The mind has long been seen as the crucible for many of our problems, such as the stories that we make up or belief patterns that have never been questioned. We can exacerbate stressful events in the way we think and react to them. We need the stillness that yoga can create so that we can see what lies beneath all the noise – our fundamental being, pure awareness.

The Path to Liberation

Experience

Yoga is an experiential practice. Yogis have been experimenting with practices, behaviours and states of consciousness to see which gets them closer to their version of liberation. Modern yogis can adopt a similar approach: explore the practices, try them out, modify them. If something doesn't work, try something else. Become aware of the results in your body, mind and spirit, and integrate them into your life.

Focus and Attention

Yoga was practised mainly by renunciant men; the emphasis was on asceticism, discipline and control, especially of the mind and the senses. This allowed awareness to come inside (*pratyahara*), away from external stimuli, which encouraged more focused concentration and enabled meditation. In our modern lives, with decreasing attention spans, practising yoga draws your attention away from distractions and is a useful skill, one that can assist you with better focus on the task at hand, as well as calming the mind.

Ethics and Behaviour

Throughout yoga's documented history, a code of ethics has been part of the path. Attitudes toward areas such as honesty (*satya*), non-possessiveness (*aparigraha*), discipline (*tapas*) and finding ease (*santosha*) are found in several yogic texts, the most famous being the *Yoga Sutras*. A key behaviour is that of non-harming (*ahimsa*) toward self and others, in thought and deed. These guidelines are seen as the first step on any yogic path, before other practices, such as postures or breathwork. Choosing a

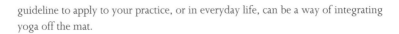

guideline to apply to your practice, or in everyday life, can be a way of integrating yoga off the mat.

Managing Energy

Yoga is also based on managing energy (*prana*) in the body, through movement to breath and meditation. We can breathe to calm the nervous system, or to raise energy up to the head (Kundalini) for a sense of open awareness. In our modern posture practice the effect on the nervous system via the fascia (see page 37) will affect our state of mind and energy levels, too. This enables us to move stuck energy in the body–mind and start to repattern our movements and thinking.

Discernment

Discernment is about sharpness of thinking. Emphasized by the Tantrics, it is crucial to the cultivation of awareness. Examples might include examining whether a particular class or style is really right for you, or whether your lifestyle is helping you. It might also mean inquiring into patterns that you have accumulated, or listening to messages from your heart and gut, which is why so many yoga practices are embodied.

Letting Be

Practices of "letting be" are found throughout yoga: surrendering to the pose, to the breath, to the universe. We are taught that we are masters of our own destiny, but you can plan and work hard and sometimes it doesn't work out and you need to walk away. Yoga means knowing when to push, and when to let go and hand over to someone or something else. You can experience this in your physical yoga: when to attempt a stronger pose or variation and when to back away.

Compassion and Curiosity

The practice of yoga is not easy to master, so compassion and curiosity are important. As yoga is experimental, we can bring curiosity toward our bodies, minds and emotions and explore what we find. We can treat ourselves kindly: for example, by taking a restorative class when we're exhausted, rather than pushing through a more vigorous practice. When we soften and open in this way, we can also expand our awareness, finding other perspectives and new possibilities.

2
HOW YOGA WORKS

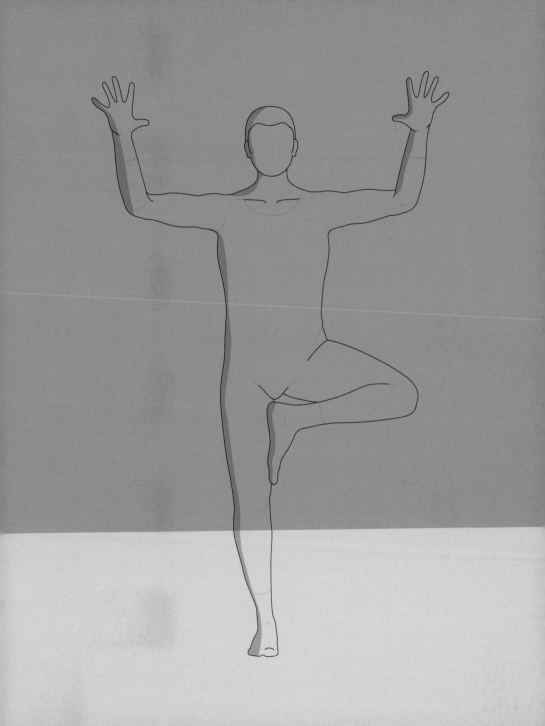

How Yoga Works

Yoga practices are a set of tools with which we can cultivate awareness. It is through this awareness that we wake up to reality and our true nature. Yoga practices also provides ways of managing that awareness, so that we can live more easily.

The main tool of this awareness is *prana* or energy. Yoga practices move *prana* in the physical, mental and emotional layers of the body, unblocking whatever has become stuck and getting us more in tune with ourselves. We will start to notice what works for us energetically in terms of food, other people, work, hobbies and nature.

Much of what yoga accomplishes is getting us to notice and then unwind patterns in the body, mind and energetic body. We do this by exploring new possibilities in our range of movement and strength, and by understanding the integrated nature of our bodies and how the different components work together. We develop greater resilience, not only physically, but also mentally and emotionally. Improved breath also helps to regulate the nervous system and move energy flows in the body.

The embodiment of breath, movement and visualization gives us a better connection to our mental and emotional states. We start to feel emotions rather than push them away, which enables us to develop a new reality. We can improve concentration and attention, and also become aware of other potential outcomes. Yoga enables us to create space around stories and beliefs, so that we can see life for what it is: we can respond to what is really going on, rather than how we would like things to be. Enhanced awareness means that we can notice more of the good in life, even in small moments.

Through deep relaxation we can nurture and reset our nervous system, and allow space for this unwinding of patterns and shifting of energy. Rest brings us to a place of greater equanimity for the challenges that greater awareness can bring.

Prana

Prana is universal energy, or life force, which is available everywhere. In the yogic energy system, prana is that which makes everything alive, from food to animals and humans. Prana is also present in buildings, rocks and plants. Everything is made up of energy, and it is all vibrating all the time. Even in modern physics this vibrational pattern has been acknowledged.

When it flows into us, prana feeds us, keeps us feeling alive and energetic. If we have too much prana outside, we can feel restless, flaky or worried. If we don't have enough prana inside, we can feel aimless, stuck or fatigued. Prana is said to flow in the nadi system of body channels (see page 247).

Our bodies are often "blocked", which means there isn't room for prana to enter or move freely inside. Many yoga practices concern clearing unwanted "stuff" from the body and freeing up blockages. You may have had the experience of something "shifting" after a yoga class. Yoga techniques are used to heat and cleanse the body of this stuff. They can also be used to cool and calm the nervous system, as well as for directing energies around the body.

In yogic terms, our system can be full of energy that is stuck in the body – emotional blockages – where feelings have not been fully processed or digested; and psychological blockages from the past, or certain beliefs that limit our potential. The chakra (energy centre) and nadi systems are used as maps to understand blockages and stuck energy, or as places where we need more energy. Traditionally yogis, or yoga experts, were moving energy in order to explore an altered state of consciousness. Today we may wish to use the practices for something simpler – for example, after a hectic day you might need to ground your energy by directing it downward. Alternatively, if you are feeling sluggish, you may wish to raise your energy more to the crown of your head.

The Physical Body

In the following sections we will look at how yoga works on our bodies, our breath, energetically and in more subtle ways, such as emotionally and mentally. Yoga has always had a link to the physical body. The earliest practices used *pranayama*, or breath control, to move *prana*, or energy, through the body to change the state of consciousness. Later came more subtle maps of the body, such as *nadis* (see page 247), *chakras* (see page 248) and *koshas*, or layers (see page 250). Hatha yogis developed postures and "cleansing" techniques to move *prana*. In the modern period, yoga has become more about movement, but the aim has never changed: how to shift energy in the body so that we can cultivate awareness and change our state.

Today we need a more obviously physical way to become embodied – feeling more deeply into, and connecting with our bodies – hence the importance of *asanas*, or yoga postures. Unfortunately, too much of our modern yoga has become about these shapes, with a focus on how to do them "properly", rather than on using them as tools to connect to ourselves physically, and then more deeply.

In this part of the book we will look at aspects of the physical body, anatomy, the brain, the nervous system and how we move, as well as at individual poses. Remember: it's all about how you find connection to your body, what you learn about it, how it moves and feels, rather than whether you can do the poses "properly". Yoga lies in the awareness that you cultivate, not in the shapes.

The Original Body

When considering the body, it helps to know where we came from, both as a life form and as individuals. Our collective and individual histories play a large role in our bone structure, our build and our tissues, and consequently in how we move through yoga poses and, more importantly, through life.

At some point in our evolution we came onto land and encountered gravity. Gravity exerts a force on the body, which it needs to resist. This resistance creates the tension needed to keep the body upright, otherwise gravity would make us a pool of sludge on the floor. Tension comes from the connective tissue supporting the bones, and from the creation of cavities in the body, such as the ribcage, abdomen and pelvis. At the same moment as we experienced gravity, we also felt oxygen in our lungs as we breathed in and out, thus developing our diaphragm as a key breathing and postural muscle. In subsequent millennia we learned to stand up, so that our head went above our heart, freeing up our upper limbs from walking, so that they could be used for other tasks.

We were built for a range of different movements. Traditionally humans were nomadic hunter-gatherers who expended energy on the hunt, then rested in small communities of about 150 people. We evolved into pastoralists and herders, with animals to look after, although usually still with semi-nomadic lifestyles. We drank the animals' milk and ate their meat, and grew bigger. With the arrival of the agricultural revolution we learned to domesticate crops and animals, so there was a constant food supply. With this came the start of the repetitive movement patterns we see today. These repetitive movement patterns have put additional tension and stress in the body, and removed strength from areas where we need it.

In post-natal development, babies start out on their backs, but then learn to be on their tummies, hold their head up, then sit up, and then roll over. They learn to move their arms to grab things, and move their legs to get traction with their feet, to start to crawl. They learn to move the pelvis under the torso to stand up. These movements are organic and intrinsic to us as humans and part of our movement in yoga is to enable the body to move back more toward its original state.

How We Move and Why It Matters

We are designed to move: to walk, run, pick things from trees above us, squat and jump. Watch a young child at play to see the range of free movement they engage in. Over time, we lose this ability and become stiffer, and lose our range of movement. Movement stems from the nervous system, because it sends commands to the muscles to move, which articulates the joints. We can strengthen these messages, and the ability of the muscles to respond, through gentle repetition and practice.

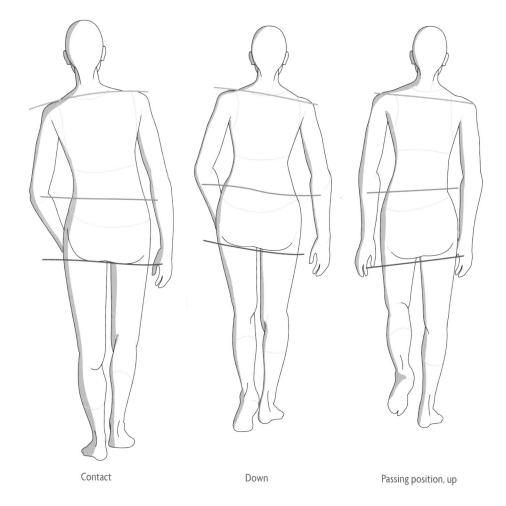

Contact   Down   Passing position, up

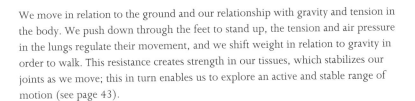

We move in relation to the ground and our relationship with gravity and tension in the body. We push down through the feet to stand up, the tension and air pressure in the lungs regulate their movement, and we shift weight in relation to gravity in order to walk. This resistance creates strength in our tissues, which stabilizes our joints as we move; this in turn enables us to explore an active and stable range of motion (see page 43).

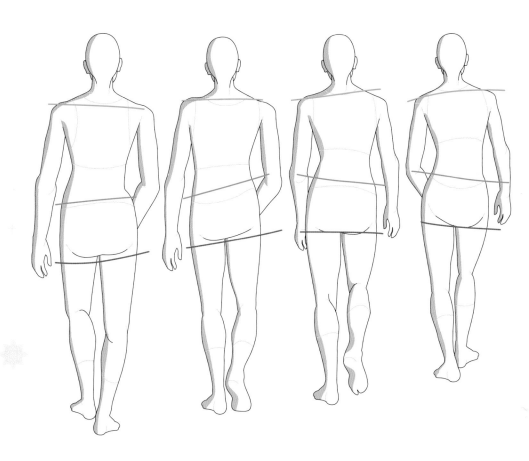

Contact   Down   Passing position, up   Contact

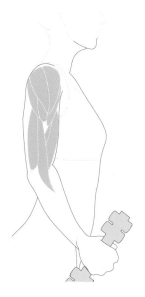

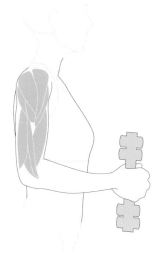

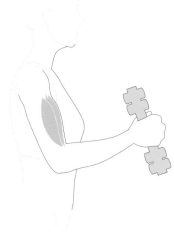

Eccentric muscle contractions:
Where a lengthening happens to
help us change position or the
angle of a joint.

Isometric muscle contractions:
These help us hold poses or hold
still with tension.

Isotonic muscle contractions:
These affect the length of a muscle
and help us move.

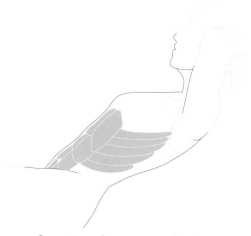

Concentric muscle contractions: Where the
muscles shorten.

Muscles work in opposite or antagonistic pairs, so that as one muscle engages, the other releases; and there are other muscles involved, especially around the joints, to help with this action.

These movements then articulate the joints so that our skeletal system responds. We use all of these types of muscle contraction in every movement, whether running or breathing, and our muscles need to perform all these movements in order to function healthily. Our joints need the muscles to move so that they have a wide range of movement and can articulate well.

Fascia

The secret ingredient is the fascia – a bandage or clingfilm-like tissue, which wraps itself around the body, from under the skin, joints and organs. We need our fascia, muscles and joints to be supple and fluid to allow freedom of movement, as this enables all their surfaces to glide against each other. The fascia will follow repetitive movements or patterns in the body, such as sitting a certain way, and will start to mould itself to this. It becomes stiff and reduces its line of movement.

The fascia needs to stay well hydrated as well as mobile. Think of when you wake up in the morning: you feel tight, stiff and achy; it feels lovely to stretch and reach and wriggle. This is the fascia feeling dehydrated and stiff from being still all night; notice how it loves to move and be unravelled.

Mobility, Stability and Flexibility

What we're looking for is the optimum ability to move, and that comes from a balance between fluidity and strength. A runner needs some stiffness and strength to stabilize the joints; however, they don't want to be too stiff, so a happy range of motion is needed to prevent overuse and injury.

Most of us do not need to stretch all the time to be more flexible. To get a better range of motion we need to move and increase our pliability. We also need to strengthen, especially in areas such as the glutes (see page 87). In our yoga practice we need not fight the body to make perfect shapes, but rather find gentle movement in and out of poses – and within poses – to allow the fascia to release and our muscles and joints to work.

Muscle Chains

The fascia or connective tissue in the body means that everything is connected to something else. When it comes to how we move, it's helpful to think about these intra-body connections and what activates through the chain of muscles. The anatomy teacher and body worker Tom Myers famously conceptualized the idea of muscle chains in his dissection work and exploration of fascia.

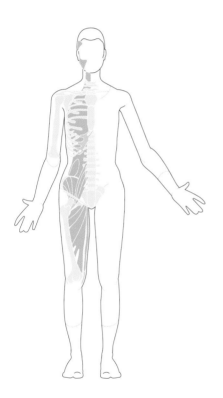
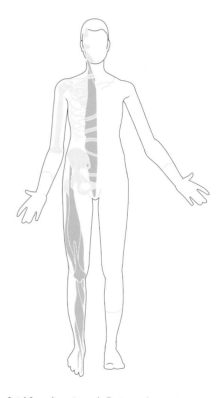

Deep front line: Our inner core, demonstrating how the "core" doesn't just mean the tummy muscles. This line is also affected by sitting, especially the adductors on the inner thighs, hip flexors and, via the diaphragm, into the throat and jaw.

Superficial front line: Controls flexion and extension of the front body, via a chain from the top of the feet, through the hips, tummy and into the sides of the throat. Crunches and sit-ups will engage this line, as will bending down to pick up something from the floor.

You will see from the pictures opposite, below and overleaf how interconnected our bodies really are, and how activating one area has a knock-on effect throughout the rest of the body. It's why we can engage our core using our hands and feet, and why sitting for long periods can have such a deleterious effect on us. Muscle chains have deep and superficial lines, which simply means that the superficial lines are closer to the skin.

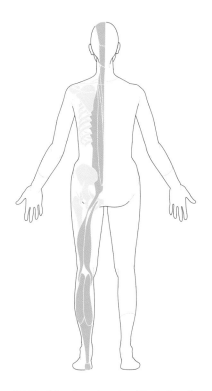

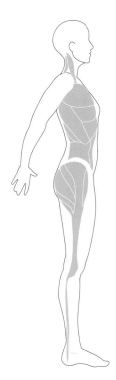

Superficial back line: From the soles of the feet, up the back legs to the erectors alongside the spine, and up the neck to cover the skull. Forward Fold (see page 98) and Down Dog (see page 148) can lengthen and mobilize this chain.

Lateral line: Controls sideways bending, using a chain from the plantar fascia in the foot, glutes and obliques.

Spiral line: Transmits cross-body forces. Try twisting in a Lunge (see pages 104 and 107).

Superficial and deep front arm lines: The front arm lines connect the hands to the chest, with a superficial line (left) supported by a deeper line (right). This is what engages during a press-up, Down Dog (see page 148) or All Fours position (see page 138).

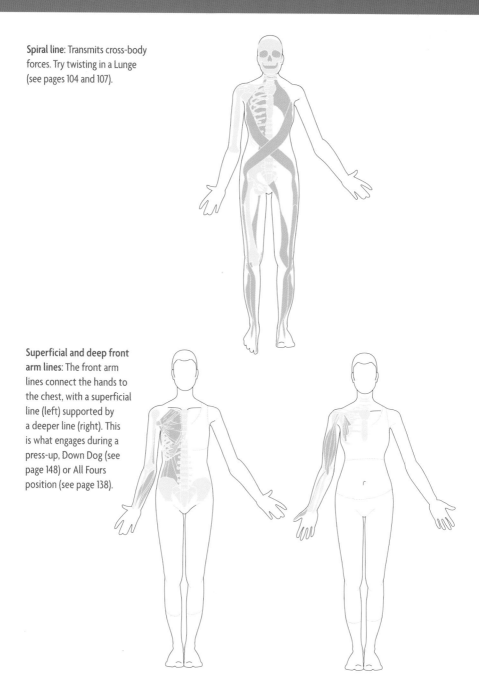

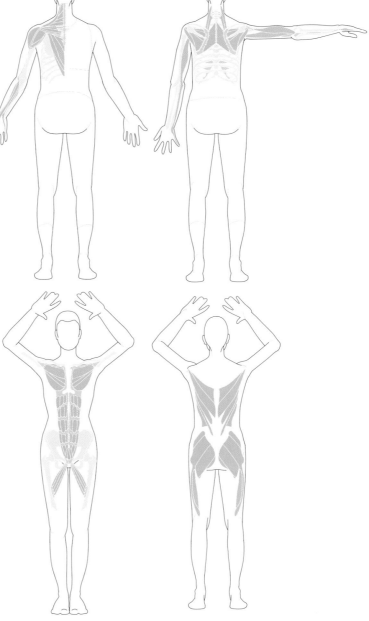

Superficial and deep back arm lines: The back arm lines connect the thumbs to the back muscles with a deep line (right) connecting to the mid-back and a superficial line (left) connecting to the upper back, neck and shoulders. (see Cow/Cat on page 144).

Front and back functional line: Sends forces from the extremities (arms and legs) through the trunk.

Understanding Patterns in the Body

We are the products of our genes and our environment, from in *utero*, to our family, our neighbourhood, education and work. All these factors lay down patterns in our bodies, which can affect our yoga practice. Although we may feel great when we start, once we have been practising for a couple of years our old patterning can make itself known in the body through strain and injury. There may be areas that never seem to get more mobile, no matter how much we work on them.

Patterning might be something as simple as inherited bone structure or sitting down all day at a computer or sawing wood repetitively with your right arm. When we are exposed to stressful situations or emotional disruptions for long periods of time, our stress response can become patterned in the body, so that when the feeling is triggered again, the same bodily response occurs. It now known that cells, tissue and neural pathways throughout our body and mind store memories, which means that past experiences have a very real physical expression.

When we are frightened or stressed, our body tenses in response. After the stressful event, the body relaxes – except when this process happens repeatedly, the muscles can stay tense by being contracted. This can impinge upon the whole body as the fascia gets frozen and the musculature is shortened. Exposure to prolonged stress or traumatic experiences are just some of the examples that can cause this patterning in the body. Eventually we may become unable to relax those muscles or parts of the body, even after years of practice. If we are unable to relax fully, the body retains some kind of alertness or vigilance: the tension in the body tells the brain that all is not well, so we may feel as though something is always "off", although we might not know what it is.

The brain is plastic and our bodies can change, so the pattern instilled in the body can be changed in the medium to long term. To repattern it, we need to move and bring awareness to our bodies as a whole. This is why taking ownership of our bodies and having an attitude of exploring each pose or kind of movement is so important. Part of our awareness cultivation in yoga is in understanding our patterns and beginning to rewire them.

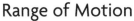

Range of Motion

"Range of motion" is our potential to move in a variety of different directions within a joint. Joints are places where two bones meet; how they move is critical for our *asana* practice and for how we get around and function in everyday life.

Some joints in the body have a greater natural range of movement, and others less range. For example, the joints in the skull bones don't move, whereas there is much more movement in the shoulder. Joints also don't work in isolation. Spinal joints have a small range of movement, but when they work together, they create considerable movement in the spine: forward, backward, sideways and rotationally.

What Affects Range of Motion?

Many people come to yoga wanting to be more flexible. Flexibility is a combination of both tissue length and suppleness, as well as range of motion in the joint.

Our joint structure is something we have limited control over. For example, having "open hips" implies a good range of external rotation, but some of this range of motion will be due to the way the head of the femur (thigh bone) is inserted into the hip socket. If it is angled toward the back, external rotation will be limited, because the femur does not have to travel far before it hits the pelvic bone. However, if the femur is inserted more toward the front of the hip socket, then greater external rotation is possible.

Some of us have ancestry from groups with larger bones, bigger bone structures and more solid builds: think Vikings, West Africans and Saxons. Others have narrower builds and smaller bones: many Asiatic groups and East Africans, for example. There is little you can do about your ancestors, except work with what you have been given!

The role of a joint in our system will also impact upon the range of motion. At the lumbar spine (lower back), forward and backward range of movement is 20 degrees, but at the thoracic (mid-back) it is 5 degrees. This is because the thoracic spine is attached to the ribcage, limiting its mobility, but giving it much greater stability and protecting the lungs and heart. Most back issues occur in the lumbar and cervical spines, due their lack of stability and greater movement – especially due to the load placed on the lumbar spine through bending, lifting and sitting.

Tissues around the joint, including muscles, ligaments, tendons and cartilage, are all involved in the movement of the joint. The condition of the tissues will have an effect on range of motion. Tight or weak muscles will limit the movement of the joint, whereas strong and lengthening muscles will be more active in movement. Weak and overly long ligaments will cause problems with stability in the joint, as there is less to hold the joint in place as it moves. Cartilage provides cushioning and stability, but also allows for movement. If it gets worn away, it can cause pain when bones meet and rub together. A classic example in yoga occurs in the knee, from kneeling on hard surfaces, where the pain is from the lack of cartilage support between the knee bones.

We can affect our range of motion in the joint structure with simple movement techniques designed to mobilize the joint. This is especially important for getting range of motion back after an injury. We can also affect range of motion by lengthening and strengthening the muscles around the joints. However, we could move and stretch for years and yet our range of motion might not change that much, if our joint structure limits it. For many students who have been practising for a long time, they are unlikely to get any bendier – and this can easily become the injury zone.

CONDITIONS AFFECTING JOINTS AND RANGE OF MOTION

Hypermobility: This is where the joints are incredibly mobile, sometimes due to a looser insertion of one bone with another. Many famous yogis were hypermobile, making it simple for them to get into some of the more contorted poses. It can be easy for hypermobile students to go into their end-range of motion, not only because of the mobility, but as hypermobility can come with a lower level of proprioception – awareness of the position of the body in space – it is harder for them to notice if they are over-extending.

Repetitive strain: This is a general term to describe the pain felt in muscles and nerves around a joint, from repeated overuse.

Yogis who do similar poses and sequences for a long time need to be aware of the impact of this on their bodies. Variety is your friend!

Arthritis: Wear and tear can cause joints to degenerate over time, resulting in painful inflammation. Such wear and tear can be magnified by pushing joints beyond their comfortable range of motion in a repeated way, although there are also other causes. However, yoga can be safe and effective for both those with osteoarthritis and rheumatoid arthritis (which is an autoimmune condition), if it is approached in a gentle way

End-Range of Motion

The end-range of motion is the furthest range we can perform with a particular joint. The end-point will be limited by either the joint structure or the tissues surrounding the joint. Many styles of yoga encourage practitioners to do *asanas* at their end-range of motion: this may feel as if you have gone as "deep" in your body as you can, and can't go any further; or it might look like your joints have "locked out".

When we come into our end-range of motion, our stress response (see page 63) is activated. The body instinctively understands that if we had to move quickly in this position, we would lack the engagement and sense of "coiled springiness" to do so. It is also at the end-range of motion that we can damage the tissues surrounding the joints, such as ligaments and tendons, as well as the joints themselves.

The problem is that deeply held poses can feel "good", either sensation-wise or in terms of a feeling of satisfaction for doing the pose "better". Sensation can be addictive, so we need more stretching and a greater range of movement to get the same feeling. Ultimately you could be in danger of going too far. If you still want to go to the end-range of motion, then it is best to visit it for one or two breaths only, then move on.

"End-range loading" is where weight is added to a joint in its end-range of motion. The force is absorbed through the joint rather than the surrounding muscles. This is very common in one-legged balancing poses such as Tree Pose (see page 111) and Warrior 3 (see page 114), and through the elbows in All Fours (see page 138). Often this occurs not only due to lack of awareness from the student that the knee joint is in its end-range, but also from a desire to find "perfect alignment". In order to load the muscle, and not the joint, the joint must be well within its range of motion, which means there will be a bend in the knee or elbow. As soon as the joint is taken out of end-range you will feel the surrounding muscles start to engage and do their job (see the exercises on pages 46–47).

End-Range Exercises

End-Range Loading

1. Standing, keep the legs dead straight, take the left leg back behind you and lower the torso into the shape of the letter T.

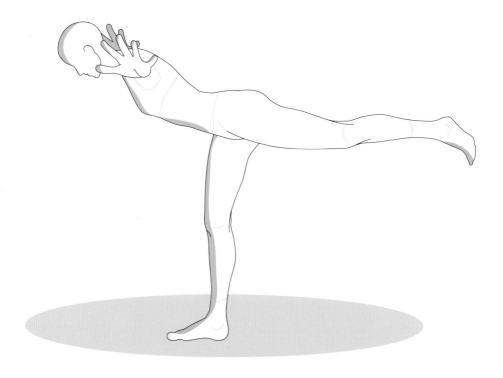

2. Notice how it feels through the straight supporting leg, especially the knee.

3. Start to bend the supporting knee; it's fine if the knee comes over the ankle a little.

4. Notice how the weight load has moved into the legs and glutes! Now the muscles are bearing the load, not the knee joint.

Find Your 60 Per Cent

Props: a strap or belt.

1. Lying on your back, bend the right knee and keep the foot planted. Take a strap or belt around the left foot and lift the leg up over the hip. The knee can be bent.

2. Ensure the left hip is grounded to the floor and shoulders and neck relaxed.

3. Move the left leg back and forward a little from the face. You are looking for maximum sensation, your deepest edge: this is your end-range of motion.

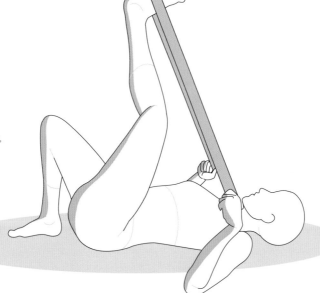

4. Allow the edge to become softer, to about 60 per cent of your maximum.

5. Stay here and breathe for 10–20 soft breaths, and notice if the sensation or edge shifts.

6. Notice any tendency to want to "push" toward your end-range of motion.

Alignment

Alignment is often thought of as the precise way to do any given pose to maximize the benefits and reduce the chance of injury. Many alignment instructions were created by the yoga teacher B K S Iyengar, and Iyengar yoga remains one of the most precision-based styles available. These instructions may not work for all body shapes. Many of these cues have now been adopted into other styles.

Many of the alignment instructions that are used in several styles of postural yoga derived from those used on young, Indian male bodies in the early to mid-20th century. Typically these young men had narrow hips and limbs and were quite mobile through the joints; they were also pretty active, and were not following the sedentary patterns of 21st-century life.

Often alignment is used for results: how to make a pose "look" better, or how to go deeper or do a "harder" version of a pose. Yoga *asanas* are a tool for cultivating awareness, releasing tension from the body and moving better. Perhaps a different way would be to find awareness of what your own body's optimal alignment might be like, using a teacher's suggestions for you to try out and see how it feels in your body.

To find an optimal alignment for your body takes practice and awareness. Here are some areas to consider when practising:

- Always stabilize the contact points you make with the floor. In standing, ensure the feet are grounded, so that the knees are supported.
- Can you explore your range of motion – for example, through arm circles or rolling up and down through the spine?
- Can you find equal space on the front and back of the body?
- Are you balanced and efficient in the body? For example, are the joints locked out or is there some "give" in them?
- Can you move in the pose? Can you wriggle, adjust or negotiate? Can you shift your weight? Can you easily move in and out of the pose?
- Don't worry about making straight lines! There are no straight lines in your body.
- How is the breath: laboured, ragged, held? These can all be examples of how the body is not in its own alignment.

Let's look now at some examples. Try the following positions and see how stable and supported your whole body feels.

Stabilize the Feet and Lower Limbs in Mountain Pose

In a standing position such as Mountain Pose (see page 97) our feet are holding up the entire body, so the lower limbs need to be stabilized.

- **Traditional**: Stand with feet together or with feet a fist-width apart, straight legs.
- **Try**: Put the feet in a place where you feel supported, with unlocked knees.

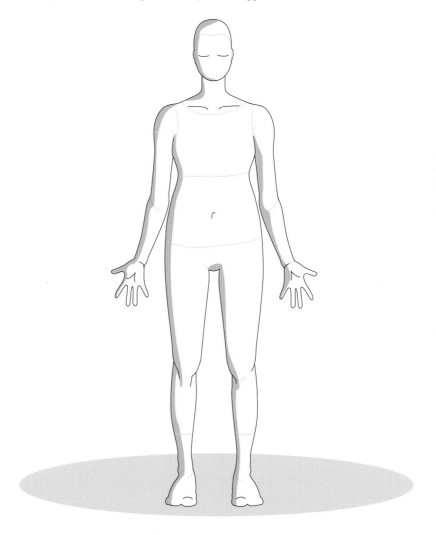

Stabilize the Knees in Lunges and Warrior 2

In a lunging position we want the front knee to be stabilized, so that our weight is supported. Stabilization of the knee actually comes from the foot being grounded.

- **Traditional**: Align the front knee over the middle front toes.
- **Try**: Bring a little more weight into the outside edge of the front foot: does the front knee feel more stable, even if it is not directly in line with the toes?

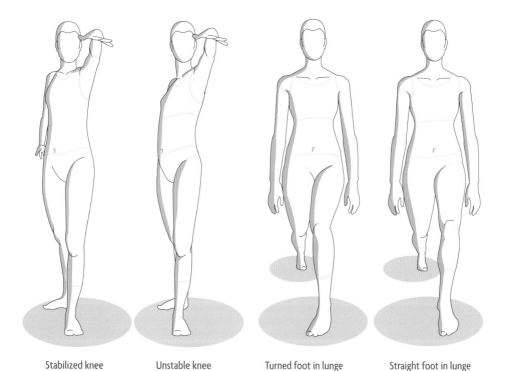

Stabilized knee   Unstable knee   Turned foot in lunge   Straight foot in lunge

Find Equal Space Front and Back

Much alignment is concerned with finding a neutral pelvis in standing positions, so that the weight is evenly distributed through the spine, pelvis, legs and feet.

- **Traditional**: Tuck or lengthen the tailbone (coccyx).
- **Try**: Notice if you can find equal space in the front and back of the pelvis, the belly and the upper torso. Tilt back and forth a little, and make small adjustments until you feel balanced, both front and back. In finding equal space, you may notice that the back feels tighter than the chest, or vice versa: these are just our everyday patterns of movement (or being sedentary!) in the body.

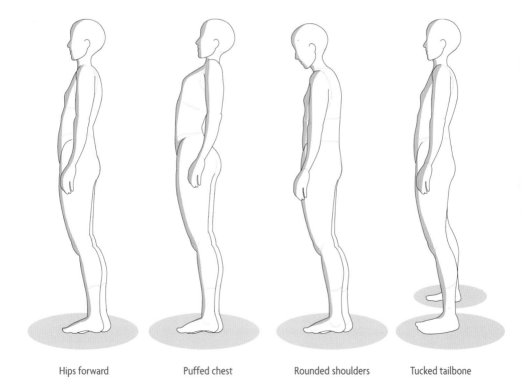

Hips forward   Puffed chest   Rounded shoulders   Tucked tailbone

Hands Support the Shoulders

When bearing weight through the hands, they support the shoulder and upper body. Hand placement can have an effect on how supported we are.

- **Traditional**: The index fingers should point forward, elbow creases point inward.
- **Try**: Come into All Fours (see page 138) and place your hands in ways that support your shoulders, but leave space around the neck: the elbows are not locked, there is some pliancy there. Experiment! Is there space across the upper back, rather than the shoulder blades dipping toward each other? As long as the weight of your shoulders and torso is supported, find what works for you.

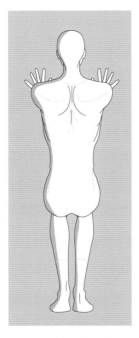

Collapsed shoulder blades

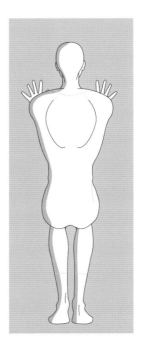

Protracted shoulder blades

Integrate Across the Back

In positions that support our body weight, we want to integrate the shoulder blades across the mid-back and fire up the muscles underneath the armpits and under the ribcage.

- **Traditional:** In All Fours (see page 138) or Down Dog (see page 148), press down the thumb and forefinger more than the rest of the hand: this activates the kinetic (muscle movement) chain to the front of the shoulders.
- **Try:** Put more weight on the little finger edge and heel of your hand, soften the elbows and notice those muscles around the side body and mid-back. Push down and see if you can feel extra space across the shoulder blade.

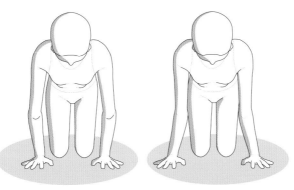

Dragging hands back   Elbows locked out

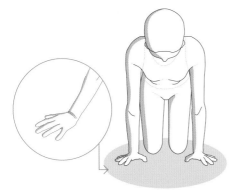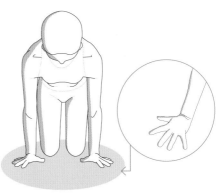

Outside edges of hands   Thumb and forefinger down

Active and Passive

In yoga we are often encouraged to stretch, go "deeper", be more flexible and stay for longer. This isn't particularly great for our bodies, especially if it's all we do, because of the difference between the effects of active engagement and passivity in the body and on the nervous system. Yoga is starting to change, to incorporate more active movement and versions of traditional poses, and these are included in this book.

Active vs Passive Range of Movement

Active range of movement (ROM) is where a joint is moved using just the muscles that surround it, without any external assistance. Passive ROM is where assistance is used, such as your hands. In the latter, the nervous system doesn't work as efficiently, as it doesn't have as much control.

Try the Passive ROM and Active ROM movements shown below and opposite. You may notice a difference between your active and passive ROM, which is known as a "neurological barrier". This is the point where the nervous system stops the active ROM because it perceives that it isn't safe, because it loses control over the

Passive ROM: Lift the knees to your chest using your hands, noticing how high up they come.

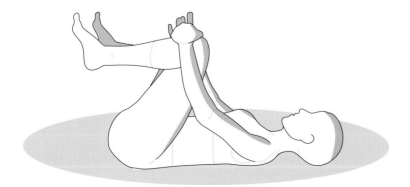

movement after this point. It may also be a perceived threat of impingement, or of locking out the joint, which the nervous system interprets as dangerous, because if our joints are locked out, we cannot move in the face of a threat.

It is not that passive ROM is bad. It can be very helpful to work on lengthening tissues and strengthening joints, if done mindfully, with intention and a judicious use of props. Careful noticing of not going beyond the end-range of movement, or staying within the 60 per cent mark, is also a good idea. In class, becoming aware of our neurological barrier and end-range of motion, and working with them, is a great way to keep the body safe and cultivate body awareness.

Passive poses are loved because they can feel like a nice stretch or sensation, and the stillness and passivity can be very calming and meditative for the nervous system. Passive poses are great at the end of class, to wind down before *Savasana* (see page 206) and for the sensation of lengthening anything that feels tight. A yin class, which is all passively held poses, is also great for lengthening and mindfulness – paying attention in the present moment – but should be part of an overall diet of movement and strengthening.

Active ROM: Lift the knees to your chest without using your hands. This is your active ROM, where the nervous system is working hard to control the movement.

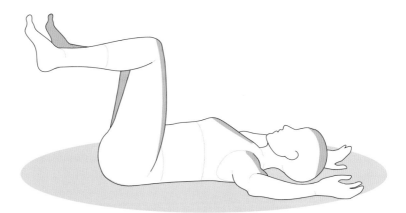

Movement and Poses

Active movement is where there is strength, control and tension involved in engaging the body in the movement or pose. This engagement means that you might not rotate as far, but you will feel more! A passive pose is where no strength is used, or where external assistance is needed.

Poses and movement can be made active in various ways:
- Engaging a particular region of the body.
- Using props to enhance tension, such as squeezing a block.
- Not using your hands to assist yourself in a particular pose.
- Making good contact to the floor or wall through the hands and feet, to engage the kinetic chain of muscles; moving slowly through transitions, or from one pose to another.

A WORD ON "STRETCHING"

Stretching is where a muscle lengthens between its origin and insertion (end) point. It feels great, and this is due to the release of compounds called opioids. Like all things that feel good, after a while we tend to need more of it to get the same experience. So we stretch more, stay for longer and use our hands, or other people, to pull us deeper. All of which can, and does, result in injury.

Research on stretching is mixed. While muscles do need to lengthen, what humans tend to need more of is strength. We often stretch things that feel tight and painful. The stretch relieves the pain – for a while – then it hurts again and we need to do more stretching. What might be more effective is to strengthen other areas that will help relieve the tightness or soreness, so that the stretch isn't needed as much.

Consulting a body worker or other professional, such as an osteopath or physiotherapist, may result in strength exercises to do at home to help rebuild your strength.

Linear vs Non-Linear Movement

Modern postural yoga's revival as a physical culture movement for young Indian men, as part of the resistance to colonial rule, provided a militaristic context. And young teenage boys need structure! Over the decades this has been transmitted to Western practitioners, where it is now the norm. We move back and forward on the mat through a Forward Fold (see page 98) or Down Dog (see page 148), make nice circles with our arms, or flex and extend the spine in Cow/Cat (see page 144). Sometimes we might rock from side to side on our backs or do a twist. We need to stay on the mat, follow the teacher's instruction and not interfere with our neighbours in a crowded room.

Linear motion is movement of an object from one place to another in a straight, or mostly straight, line. However, the body can also move in a non-linear way. Non-linear motion refers to any non straight-line movement with changing direction: for example, turning to face the other end of the mat, rotating the arm as you make circles or finding spirals through the spine. This type of movement will engage more of the whole body and has a very different effect on the nervous system. When we don't move in straight lines, new neural pathways are needed to explore the new movement. At the same time the freedom of not needing to stay in a box can be very liberating for body and mind. Non-linear movement can also increase our range of motion, by bringing in new movements and directions and challenging the joints and tissues to move in a novel but safe way.

In the Poses section of this book (see pages 96–209), options will be given both to move in a traditional linear way and to explore non-linear variations, too. There are exercises to get you started on pages 58–59.

Linear Movement Exercises

Linear Arm Circles

1. In All Fours (see page 138), slowly
make arm circles.

2. Notice how your arm can go
back and forward.

3. Notice how any restrictions in
the shoulder will mean that the
arm might have to move a little:
that's okay.

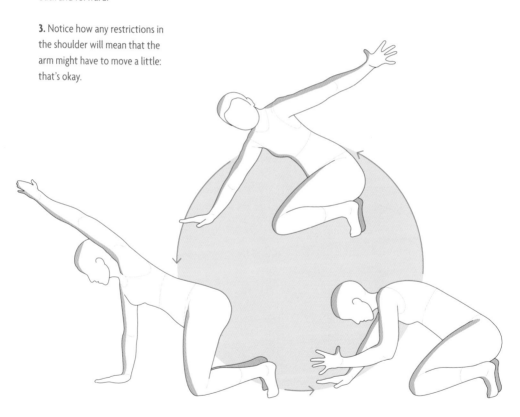

Non-Linear Arm Circles

1. Now turn the palm to face different directions as you make circles.

2. Notice where you have to turn back, or bend the arm, or move the spine.

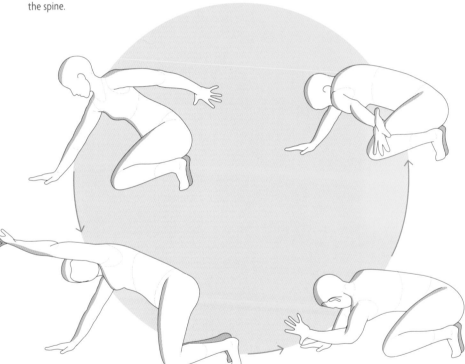

3. Imagine you are balancing a cup of tea in your hand: what kind of movements can you make with the arm, without dropping the tea?

4. Make wider circles, bringing the arm in front or out to the side.

5. Keep making circles: there is nowhere to get to here – just explore!

The Nervous System

For most practitioners the feelings of relaxation, calmness, a sense of flow, an increase in energy and other related outcomes are some of the main reasons for doing yoga. What causes this response is down to how our yoga practice affects the nervous system. In the past, the outcomes of yoga were purely experiential. Now we understand what is happening in the body on a physiological basis, too.

The nervous system is complex and not yet fully understood. What is included here just scratches the surface, and research into how the nervous system works and its implications is being developed all the time.

The nervous system comprises several main sections:
- **Central Nervous System:** the brain and spine.
- **Peripheral Nervous System:** the nervous system outside the brain and spine.
- **Autonomic Nervous System:** part of the peripheral system, the Autonomic Nervous System (ANS) is responsible for body functions that are not consciously directed, such as breathing.
- **Enteric Nervous System:** part of the ANS, this is the nervous system of the gut.

Motor and Sensory Nerves

We have motor and sensory nerves in the body, and both are needed for movement. Motor nerves coordinate the muscles to achieve movement, but without the sensory muscles we wouldn't know where the muscles or body parts are. When you wake up in the dark, you know where your arms are without looking at them, via your sensory nerves. This is called proprioception, and it's needed a lot in yoga – for example, when stepping back into a lunge. Yoga can improve our proprioception, as the repetition strengthens the sensory-nerve messaging to the brain.

Our nervous system is also integral to how aware we are of messages, sensations and feelings inside the body: everything from hunger, to needing the toilet, to emotions. This is called interoception. Yoga can also improve this inner awareness, especially through breathwork, visualization and meditation. The whole subtle body of yoga (see page 246) can be seen as exercises in interoception – such as using the model of the *chakra* energy circles in the body to check in with our stored emotions (see page 248–249).

Sensory nerves lie deep in the fascia. This explains how we can "breathe" into the back of the legs, even if our lungs are not actually there. Our sensory nerves and visualization create a powerful ability to feel. These sensory nerves are also why stretching can feel so good, especially in areas that seem "tight". Certain parts of the body have more nerve endings, such as the soles of the feet and the hands. This is so that contact with the ground, or things we pick up, can set off a kinetic chain through the body, so that we can move and respond using the motor nerves. In addition, sensory nerves tell us how much grip to use or how much pressure to hold a glass with.

Motor nerves are found in the muscles and joints. To learn new movements, our nervous system has to learn to coordinate the muscles to move the joints to work in a certain way: the so-called "mind–muscle connection". This motor learning uses practice, repetition and feedback, which is why repeating postures and sequences can be beneficial when learning. The neural pathways of the specific mind–muscle connection strengthen, and the movement becomes faster and more efficient.

The body and mind also love variety, so once a particular movement is working, it is good to change it up. The poses and sequences in this book give lots of options to add variety so that even more neural pathways can be developed and new motor learning generated!

The Autonomic Nervous System

The Autonomic Nervous System controls the unconscious processes in the body: breathing, gut function, heart rate and others. Specifically with yoga and meditation, the ANS manages our Sympathetic Nervous System (SNS) and Parasympathetic Nervous System (PNS), which govern our response to stress.

The system developed so that when we experienced a threat to our person, our SNS – our fight-or-flight mode – would switch on. When activated, our body prepares to fight the aggressor, to run away or to freeze. All the body's resources will be directed to aid this purpose, and any other processes will be downgraded or switched off; for example, blood will flow to the major muscle groups to enable us to fight or run. The body desperately wants to return to balance, or homeostasis, so it wants the threat to be resolved: by escaping or hiding. The system was designed for short-term, emergency use, whereby homeostasis would be resumed shortly.

Today most threats are to our identity and self-concept: the fear of being not good enough at work; not liked by our friends; not getting all of our to-do list done plus being concerned for others. It doesn't matter if the threat is physical or otherwise; if it is real or imagined, such as worrying about the future – the body reacts by activating the fight-or-flight system. Unlike in the distant past, homeostasis is difficult to find for many of us. Our SNS can be triggered by various things throughout the day, such as the alarm clock, caffeine, problems at work or getting children ready for bed. Even our social lives are heavily scheduled, with little downtime. Experiencing some stress is good for us: it brings a sense of vitality and improves our resilience; but too much over the long term can be devastating for both physical and mental health.

Being in fight-or-flight mode, with the body full of adrenaline, is incredibly tiring. Yoga works by activating the PNS, which is the rest-and-digest, tend-and-befriend model. The PNS is activated by stimulating the vagus nerve, which is the main switch of the PNS; it is a long, winding nerve that travels from the gut to the brainstem, passing by the major internal organs and the diaphragm. When we practise abdominal, diaphragmatic or yogic breathing, we massage the vagus nerve, improving its tone, or its ability to tell the brain that all is well – it's time to relax. That is why so many yoga classes start with the practice of connecting to the breath: it tells the brain it's okay to switch to rest-and-digest mode.

"Polyvagal theory" has shown that there are, however, two sides or branches to our vagal nerve: one an ancient system that all vertebrates have, and one that only more sophisticated mammals – including humans – have evolved. The earlier branch switches on the collapsed state, or "playing dead": a simple way to avoid threats, which conserves our energy. The more evolved branch regulates stress by allowing us to socialize and find support from family and friends. It triggers the release of oxytocin, the chemical of connection, which makes us feel good around loved ones. These social elements are a great way to help us manage the stress in our lives. It is helpful to notice what your tendencies are: do you shut down and avoid people, when stressed, or do you reach out? This might not necessarily be driven by your personality, and could have more to do with the strength of the more evolved branch of your vagus nerve.

There is a complicated and, as yet, not fully understood relationship between the muscular–fascia system, the nervous system and its effects on our stress levels, hormone levels, perception of pain, experience of emotions and overall wellbeing. This embodiment of stress is why movement and body workers are so crucial to our ability to manage our stress levels: we need to move, to release tension and calm the nervous system in order to help calm the mind. Our thoughts have a real impact on our perception of the world: the body doesn't know what is real or imagined, so anxious thoughts can easily trigger a stress response in the body, which is perceived as tension by an anxious mind, generating more anxious thoughts. Yoga and meditation can help, by calming the body and mind, but for more severe cases a doctor must be consulted for additional resources.

Depending on the style of yoga, some part of a yoga class might stimulate the SNS – usually the more vigorous sequences or stronger poses. Many of us are over-adrenalized, and all that adrenaline has to go somewhere, so a flow practice can be useful, with a long relaxation at the end. If we are exhausted, then yin or restorative yoga (see page 15) or a meditation class may be best.

Classes should end with some passive or restorative poses, maybe some breathing or meditation, and then the all-important *Savasana* (see page 206). This is where the nervous system and the physical body restore themselves, but it's also where they process the movements you have been practising, so the neural pathways can learn and grow.

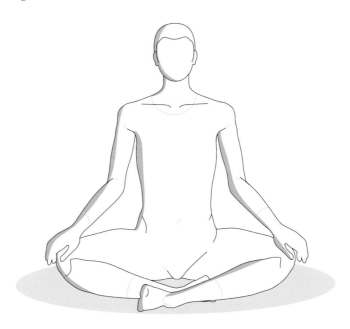

How Yoga Impacts Upon the Brain

We now know that yoga and meditation have profound effects on the structure and activity of the brain. In structural terms, we can simplify the brain's complex make-up into three parts. This is known as the **Triune Brain Theory**.

- **The reptilian brain:** the oldest part of the brain, four million years old. It is associated with survival and our fight-or-flight response – not just our physical safety, but also threats to our identity. It is located in the brainstem and cerebellum, and governs much of what we do on autopilot.
- **The mammalian brain:** the next oldest part, about 250 million years old. This is where we learned to care for our offspring, and is associated with emotions, memories and habits. It is related to feelings of warmth and connection.
- **The human brain:** the newest part, about 500,000 years old. It is located in the neocortex, the outer layer of the brain, and governs language, abstract thought, imagination and consciousness. In this way it is used for reasoning, rational thought, self-control and awareness.

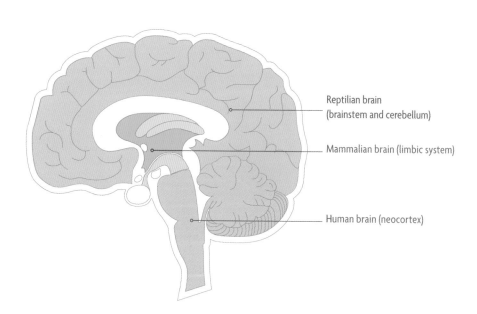

Reptilian brain
(brainstem and cerebellum)

Mammalian brain (limbic system)

Human brain (neocortex)

One of the issues we humans have is that we have "three brains in one", often sending competing messages. On receiving an angry email from a friend, our reptilian brain can go into "threat" mode, causing us to be defensive and reactive to the criticism. Our neocortex, which is in charge of self-regulation, may just be able to communicate that reacting in this way is not a great idea; perhaps it would be better to take a deep breath and consider our friend's perspective. Meanwhile, our mammalian brain may even remember the warm, close feelings we get from the friend, when things are going well. So which brain wins? How do we respond?

Bringing the Neocortex "Online"

Yoga, meditation and mindfulness work by stimulating the neocortex, bringing about greater self-regulation and an ability to respond, not react. It is not that we don't get a flush of anger as emotion surges through our body, and negative thoughts and unpleasant feelings. But yoga practice allows us to be calm and to check in with ourselves, and not lash out in a habitual or automatic way.

Structurally, yoga and meditation cause several changes in the brain. Richard Davidson at the Center for Healthy Minds at the University of Wisconsin has found that regular meditation practice activates the left prefrontal cortex, at the front of the head, associated with increased feelings of love, kindliness, curiosity and acceptance. Meditation is also said to help the three brains work better together, by improving the synchronization of the left and right hemispheres. Other structural changes include an increase in grey matter in the cortex, which improves focus and attention; and even more folds in the brain, leading to better processing speed. There is said to be reduction of activity in the amygdala, our fear centre, and an increase in the hippocampus, the centre of learning.

There are also chemicals being released in and from the brain, which greatly affect how we think, feel and behave. Yoga and meditation change the levels of various chemicals, causing an overall effect of reduced stress and greater calm – for example, reducing cortisol and adrenaline, as part of the fight-or-flight response; and increasing the feel-good chemicals serotonin and oxytocin.

Neural Pathways: "What Fires Together, Wires Together"

There are more than 100 billion neurons in the brain that form connections, leading to neural pathways. These pathways relate to thoughts, behaviours, movements, emotions, memories and many other functions. Although there are countless ways for the neurons to connect, the neurons that we activate are the ones that will build a pathway. This is why repeated thoughts and actions can become habitual patterns in the mind and body.

Some of these neural pathways are like a wide motorway, with traffic flowing freely, often without any conscious input from us at all. Others are more like overgrown tracks through the backwoods. To improve these neural pathways will take practice and conscious effort on our part.

The concept of neuroplasticity shows that while we used to think the brain was fixed in childhood and couldn't change, we now know that it can and does change, with the right inputs. Repeating actions helps us learn to sit and meditate, or how to do a particular pose. However, changing our sequence, style or teacher is also important, so that we fire up even more new neural pathways. Yoga also improves levels of brain-derived neurotrophic factor, a protein that is needed for neuron health and neuroplasticity.

Yoga philosophy understood the idea of patterns of behaviour, thoughts and emotions getting stuck neurologically in the body. Today we would call these habitual neural pathways our "conditioning", but the yogis called them *samskaras*. One of the goals of yoga is to unwind our *samskaras* though our practice. In modern terms, we need to rewire our brains!

Brain Waves

The neurological connections described above create brain waves: as the neurons communicate, they produce synchronized electrical pulses. These pulses lie at the root of all our thoughts, emotions, dreams and actions. The ability to manage our brain waves can be important: brain-wave activity runs the full spectrum from deep sleep to problem-solving, but we increasingly spend more time in "doing" activities, rarely giving our brains and nervous system a rest. Yoga works by switching us from "doing" brain waves into the slower and deeper frequencies associated with rest, repair, awareness and deep knowing. The descriptions in the chart opposite are broad ones, because the reality is far more complex: brain waves can reflect differently, depending on which location in the brain they occur.

TYPES OF BRAINWAVE

Brainwave	Pattern	Frequency	Description	Yoga practices	How yoga works
Gamma		40–99 Hz	High-speed cognitive processing. Linked to "consciousness".	Deep meditation for long periods/ years of practice.	Prolonged meditation allows access to improved levels of awareness.
Beta		13–39 Hz	Focus, problem-solving, thinking, "doing mode", wide awake. Cannot be sustained indefinitely, as prolonged beta-activity leads to exhaustion and anxiety.	Our usual state! Learning a new pose or taking a much more difficult class might need beta waves to "think" our way through the sequence.	Yoga moves us out of beta waves and gives us time to rest.
Alpha		8–12 Hz	Relaxed "being mode", internally focused and self-reflective.	Gentle flow, restorative yoga, yin yoga, mindfulness meditation.	Integrating body and mind. Good before exams, as it increases accelerated learning.
Delta		0.5–3.5 Hz	Deep sleep and deep relaxation.	Yoga Nidra (see page 263).	Improved sleep, ability to get to sleep; better repair at night.
Theta		4–7.5 Hz	Relaxed, but deeply aware. Access to the subconscious. Creative problem-solving. Lucid dreaming.	Yoga Nidra (see page 263), deep meditation.	Meditation allows us to access the subconscious, by quietening the thinking mind so that we can go beyond it.

How Yoga Helps Manage Pain

Many people come to yoga – and increasingly are directed to yoga classes
by their doctors – because of pain. Pain may be both physical and mental/
emotional. In this section we will consider how yoga can help with physical
pain; and in the next section, how yoga helps with mental health.

Pain is an important messenger: it tells us that we need to take action to resolve a
problem. However, we tend to think of pain as "bad", and even the thought of pain
and discomfort as bad. This approach works when it concerns acute pain: short-
lived, even if strong in sensation, such as shutting your finger in a drawer. When
dealing with chronic, long-term pain, however, this approach isn't always helpful.
Pain becomes chronic when it lingers beyond about three months without healing.
Chronic pain costs a lot in terms of individual suffering, but also costs to society,
in terms of treatment and lost productivity.

When in pain, we often want something "to be done" to make it go away. An issue
with long-term chronic pain is that there is often no observable cause and it's
unclear what can "done" to make the pain go away. The nervous system doesn't
work directly – pain messages do not travel in direct and exclusive pathways to the
brain. Sensory impulses originating in the body are sent to the brain, where they
are interpreted as pain; however, the amount of pain does not relate to the amount
of tissue damage. This doesn't mean that pain is imagined or isn't real; it's just that
your brain constructs your experience of pain as it does with any other event. This
opens up the possibility that mental practices, such as meditation, could help with
the experience of pain.

Our perception of an event or sensation is linked to our Autonomic Nervous System
(see page 61). If we experience pain and have negative thoughts about it, this can
activate our fight-or-flight response: the brain perceives the pain as a threat, releases
cortisol and adrenaline and increases tension in the body. The increased tension
and threat perception can make the experience of pain worse. The worsening
experience triggers the threat perception again, and so the cycle continues.

Yoga, including gentle *asanas*, slow movements, regulated breathing and meditation,
can help to activate the Parasympathetic Nervous System (see page 61). When the
PNS is switched on, it sends a message to the brain that all is well. The brain then
perceives any events or sensations as more friendly, thus reducing our perception of
pain. Research shows that just four 20-minute mindfulness meditation classes can
improve the experience of pain; the study demonstrated that the parts of the brain

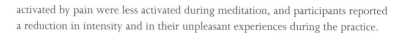

activated by pain were less activated during meditation, and participants reported a reduction in intensity and in their unpleasant experiences during the practice.

With acute pain, rest is usually advised; however, with chronic pain, rest might not be needed, as there may be no obvious trauma or injury to heal. Movement might actually work better instead. It can also help to reduce any physical inflammation. Gentle movement and *asanas* can relieve tension, which the brain may interpret as a reduction in possible threats and may change the perception of pain.

The "gate-control theory" of pain may also explain why *asanas* and movement can help with our experience of pain. This theory proposes that activation of non-pain-signalling nerves can interfere with signs from pain fibres. The non-pain nerves close a gate to the pain signals in the spinal cord, inhibiting pain. When doing yoga postures, the sensations in the body of these movements can act as a gate to pain messages, stopping them from being received by the brain: instead the brain notices the pleasant feelings coming from the *asanas*.

Listening to pain includes making sensible decisions about obtaining medical interventions when they are needed. Yoga, mindfulness and meditation are not replacements for medication and therapy, where required.

How Yoga Works with Mental Health

Gentle movement, moderate exercise and mindfulness are common prescriptions for managing our mental health. This has made yoga popular as a mental-health resource, with students reporting feeling more relaxed and less stressed and having better sleep after practising. The eight-week Mindfulness-Based Stress Reduction course developed by Jon Kabat-Zinn in the early 1980s, and now used worldwide, has evidenced reduced pain perception, anxiety and stress-related symptoms, following completion of the course.

When we move, we can affect positive changes in the body involving pain levels, mobility and physical strength, which can affect our mood and behaviour. Stretching and gentle movement release endorphins and opioids, which improve our mood and outlook. Yoga also switches us into the Parasympathetic Nervous System (see page 61), which affects anxiety and depressive symptoms by helping us relax or seek out social support. Gentle movement is also a mild stimulant, which can be energizing for those who are feeling lethargic or stuck.

Through movement, breathwork and visualization, yoga can take you away from the mind and create greater space around thoughts and mind-created suffering. This space helps with understanding reality, getting to see what is true for us, rather than the stories we hold; it gives us a chance to investigate our beliefs and patterns to see if they still serve us. When we create this new perspective, we may feel less controlled by the mind and become less reactive to its suggestions. Reducing our reactivity can allow for greater ease in dealing with whatever life throws at us, good or bad.

Mental-health issues such as stress, depression and anxiety can be so overwhelming that we only manage to deal with their symptoms, and these mask what is happening underneath. Sometimes this is for good reason: perhaps we are not ready to face our deep emotions, or they are too big or frightening to manage. Anxiety and depression can be seen as the opposite of the stress-response dial, with depression as shutdown, and anxiety as fight-or-flight: both are ways of dealing with threats and fear, even when that fear comprises past events that have stored themselves in our system. Yoga gets us in touch with our feelings by reducing the impact of anxiety and depression, so that we might be able to feel what is happening beneath these conditions.

Yoga opens us up and allows energy to shift. It enables us to feel stronger both physically and mentally, but also makes us softer: more relaxed and open. We become better equipped to manage the symptoms of anxiety and depression, so that we can then start to experience our true emotions; but yoga also brings us equanimity, so that we can process and digest what arises in us. This results in an improved connection throughout: with our bodies, with our emotions and mental states, and ultimately with ourselves. Yoga opens the cage around the heart, which so many of us – including me – have built as a form of protection. It is the deep knowing that comes from opening the heart that is central to the practice of yoga, but this connection can only come as part of a gentle, safe management of the thoughts and patterns we have created or inherited that prevent us from accessing it.

Yoga and Trauma

In recent years there has been an increase in awareness of the effects of yoga on those who have experienced some form of trauma. While yoga has many practices that can be beneficial, care must be taken that techniques do not do more harm. Examples can range from overwhelming the nervous system into fight-or-flight mode, or causing the nervous system to shut down. No practice or technique is perfect or suitable for everyone all the time. The real yoga is in noticing if something is helping you: if a technique is making you feel worse, it is not your fault, and you should stop and take time to centre. Even if a teacher is encouraging you to continue, your own experience is always more important.

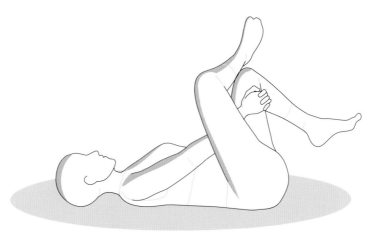

Anatomy

Understanding how our bodies are constructed and how they move will go a long way toward understanding how the yoga poses work and how they feel for us. We all have our own specific anatomy, which is based on both genetics and environment: some of it we can control, but much of it we have little or no influence over.

As we have seen, much of what we practise as modern postural yoga was designed by Indian men for other Indian men with specific lifestyles. Yogis are often thought of as being very flexible and bendy, but to a large degree this is a function of their bone structure and genetics. Yoga poses are available to all, regardless of our background, but may need modifying for those of us who lack natural mobility.

The way anatomy is taught doesn't always help us fully understand the body. In order to make a picture of muscles or bones, you have to cut something away. But the body is not built like that – there is no separation of tissues from your skin down to your bones, and into your cells: everything is connected, nothing is isolated. Moreover, anatomy often considers the body when it is static, even though many forms of yoga today are dynamic. This means that we move in the poses, and especially in transition between the poses. A lot of attention is paid to how to make the shape, but not so much to how to move in order to get there. Hopefully some of the pointers in this section will give an idea of a moving anatomy.

We will review general anatomy as it relates to our yoga practice. It is hard to separate the different parts of the body, all of which are designed to move as one integrated whole, but this breakdown will allow us to focus on the points required for our practice.

The Upper Body

The shoulder is the most mobile joint in the body and requires stability so that it doesn't get injured. The shoulder joint is composed of the head of the humerus (arm bone) sitting in a shallow ball-and-socket joint, surrounded by a complex network of muscles and ligaments.

The arm is supported by the serratus anterior muscle, which operates almost like a spring below the arm. Shoulder and neck pain can often be the result of overusing the shoulders/neck in arm movements, instead of using the serratus. During weight-bearing poses it is important to ensure that the serratus and the armpits are engaged, rather than having too much work done in the shoulder.

Shoulder Blades

Attached to the shoulder, and sitting on the back of the ribcage, are the scapulas or shoulder blades. Seventeen muscles connect to your shoulder blades and help to move your arms. Integration of the shoulder blades on the back and into the shoulder and arms is crucial for moving well. Long periods spent reaching forward to a keyboard or other device causes the scapulas to lose their integration. The serratus anterior and latissimus dorsi muscles on the back play an important role in stabilizing the shoulder blades.

Hands

Our hands provide essential functions, such as complex thumb and finger movements. In weight-bearing poses it is the connection of the hands to the ground that fires up the strong core and back muscles to support our weight. Actively using the trunk muscles will relieve pressure on the joints that are further away from us, such as the shoulder and wrist.

Wrists

Our wrists are delicate joints, providing mobility, but not a lot of stability. When we are at a keyboard, the wrists are extended, and this action is repeated in poses such as All Fours (see page 138) and Planks (see pages 132–137), with weight put through the joint. Constant scrolling, swiping and texting require repetitive finger movements, which also strain the wrist. To relieve the wrists it is important to find the correct hand engagement to fire up the muscles of the trunk.

Neck

The neck has the most mobility of all areas of the spine, being able to rotate, flex and extend in all directions, which comes at the cost of stability. Sitting and deskwork can over-stretch the back of the neck, from the connection with the shoulders to that with the base of the skull. The front of the neck and throat can become constricted and tight.

In practice you can simply turn the head or roll the chin gently in each pose to ensure that the neck is free, and find a comfortable place to rest your gaze.

Face

When the jaw is clenched or tense, the nerves pick up this message and relay it to our brain, as 80 per cent of our nerves run through the jaw. Gently releasing the jaw by moving it from side to side, opening the mouth wide and relaxing it, can feel useful. Swallowing deeply and deliberately can let the throat relax, too.

We can also soften the spot between the brows and allow the eyebrows to move away from each other. When we're stressed, our vision narrows to focus on the perceived threat, so relaxing the eye area sends an "all is well" signal to the brain.

Exercises for the Upper Body

Hands and Shoulder Connection

We can find integration and stability across the upper back with this exercise, which releases pressure on the shoulders and neck.

Props: a block or book.

1. Sitting on the floor or on a chair, take a block or book between the palms of the hands and lift it above your head.

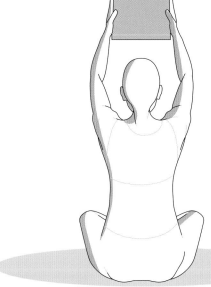

2. Squeeze the block between the hands, and notice the kinetic chain up the arms into the muscles underneath the shoulder blades.

3. See if you can keep this engagement and slowly turn from side to side.

4. If you feel this in your neck or shoulder tops, stop, rest and try again.

Shoulder-Blade Integration

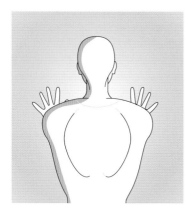

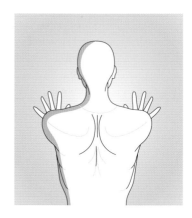

1. In All Fours (see page 138), keep the elbows soft and find a slight dragging back/pushing away movement with the hands (see Hands Support the Shoulders, page 52). Notice the movement of the shoulder blades across your back as you do this.

2. We are looking for a slight protraction (pushing apart) of the shoulder blades which will come from pushing the hands down, but not so much that the back rounds.

3. You can test your integration by hovering the knees off the ground in Tiger Plank (see page 137) or stepping back to Full Side Plank (see page 136).

Finding Armpits, Not Shoulders

1. In All Fours (see page 138), find the outside edge/heel of the hands and try to draw them slightly back toward you. This will engage the serratus and other muscles around the side body and armpit, and will allow space to occur at the top of the shoulders. Once you are comfortable with this, see if you can practise it with the knees off the ground in a Plank pose (see pages 132–137).

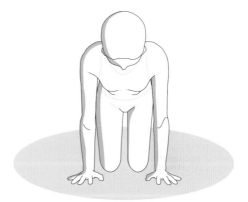

The Back

The spine is a long column of vertebrae stacked on top of each other, cushioned by discs filled with fluid. The spine is constructed in an S shape, which enables the body to manage the effects of gravity (see page 33). Each vertebra is a joint that affects the spine's movement. Most vertebrae cannot move very far on their own, but together they can create a considerable range of movement, as you can see from the table below.

SPINAL RANGE OF MOTION

Part of the spine	Also known as	Flexion/extension (bending forward and backward)	Lateral flexion (bending sideways)	Rotation
Cervical (C1–C7)	The neck.	Up to 20 degrees.	Up to 10 degrees (except C1–C2, which are 0).	Up to 47 degrees!
Thoracic (T1–T12)	The ribs.	T12: up to 20 degrees; T11–T2: decreases from 20 degrees to 5 degrees; T1: 5 degrees.	Up to 5–7 degrees.	T1: up to 8 degrees; T2–T10: decreases from 8 degrees to 5 degrees; T11–L1: less than 5 degrees.
Lumbar (L1–L5)	The waist.	Up to 20 degrees.	Up to 8 degrees.	L1–L4: Less than 5 degrees; L5/S1: 5 degrees.
Sacrum	The pelvis.	Vertebrae are fused, so there is limited movement.		
Coccyx	The tailbone.	Vertebrae are fused, so there is limited movement.		

The neck, or cervical spine, has a lot of movement, but it's also the least stable area, meaning that it is easy to injure. The thoracic spine is where the spine is attached to the ribcage; this attachment limits the range of movement. The lumbar spine, or the waist, has a considerable range of forward and backward bending, but limited rotation; this area particularly dislikes movements that combine forward/backward bending with a rotation, such as getting in and out of a car.

When we fold forward, the discs in the affected vertebrae will be pushed backward. Too much pushing can lead to herniation, where the discs bulge out between the vertebrae; if the bulging disc is pushing on a nerve in the spine, it can cause a lot of pain.

Overnight the discs get dehydrated from lying down, so in the morning they are full of water. This can impact upon your range of movement, which is why some people find yoga practice first thing more restricted than practice later on in the afternoon.

Most of us sit for long periods of the day: desk-bound jobs, driving or commuting by train. Our work is always in front us, whether it's carpentry, writing, washing up or playing with children. This creates what Dr Garrett Neill, a yoga teacher and chiropractor, called the Human Cashew Posture.

When we sit for long periods, this creates rounded shoulders, lengthened back muscles and stretched glutes and hips. There are three parallel erector muscles running from the pelvis to the ribs and base of the skull that can become over-long, losing their ability to function as stabilizers for the spine. On the front of the body, the hip flexors are tightened, and there is little room in the chest and belly to breathe, and no tone or muscular engagement in the torso.

Exercises for the Back

Thoracic Twist

The thoracic spine is meant to rotate, and the more it can do so, the greater the pressure relieved on the lumbar spine, decreasing possible lower-back pain. The Stronger Abdominal Twist (see page 200) can work, but also try this.

1. Stand tall with Cactus Arms (see page 179) in front of a mirror.

2. Rotate to the left through the thoracic spine, but ensure the hips stay still.

3. Rotate to the other side.

4. Move slowly at first, and watch in the mirror to make sure the hips don't move.

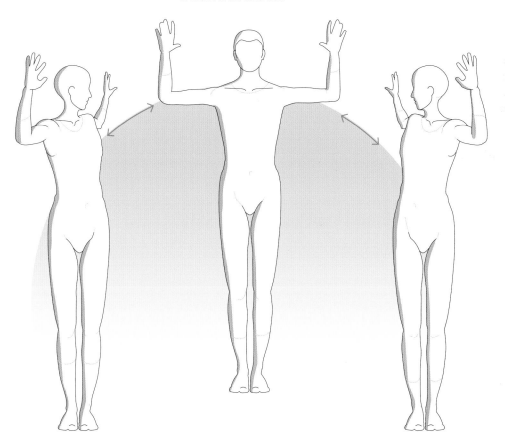

Back Extensions

This exercise adds tension and engagement into the back to counteract over-stretching from sitting.

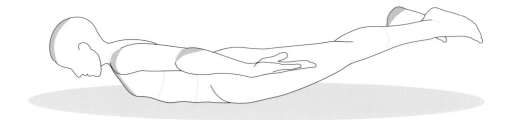

1. Lie on your front. Feel into the muscles around your mid-back, just underneath the shoulder blades: these are the muscles you are going to activate.

2. Using the mid-back, lift the head, shoulders and collarbones off the mat. If it is comfortable, you can lift the legs. Do not over-squeeze your buttocks. Exhale to come down.

3. You can also use Cactus Arms (see page 179) or Superman Arms (see page 143) in this pose. Ensure the neck remains relaxed.

LOWER-BACK PAIN – OR IS IT THE SI JOINT?

The sacroiliac (SI) joint is where the pelvis and spine meet and has very little movement. A lot of "lower-back pain" is actually occurring here, and the lumbar/SI region is very susceptible.

In side reaches, spiral reaches and seated twists, always make sure that you move your hips and pelvis with you. Be mindful of movements that involve reaching and twisting, especially with the added load

of a shopping bag. If you do experience SI joint pain, some gentle movement may help, but avoid strong *asana* practice until the issue has subsided; and if it doesn't subside, see a registered osteopath or physiotherapist for advice.

The Core

Whenever "the core" is mentioned, what most commonly springs to mind is six-pack abs. But the core is far more complicated and important than mere aesthetics.

Structurally, the ribcage and the pelvis are connected joint-wise only by the spine. The cavity in between holds vital organs, such as the liver, stomach, kidneys, pancreas and intestines. Our main breathing muscle, the diaphragm, sits under the ribs on top of these organs. Regulating the load on this cavity, and ensuring happy alignment between the ribcage and the pelvis below, is a key role for the core. Strength in the core section of the body also reduces overwork on our extremities, such as the wrists. When working well, our core enables us to make a full range of movements across the body, such as running, jumping, reaching and lifting.

At the top sits the diaphragm; down the sides are the obliques; at the bottom is the pelvic floor; at the back are various back muscles, such as the erectors, and at the front is the transverse abdominis muscle, as well as the infamous rectus abdominis (those six-pack muscles). Understanding what they all do, and how they interrelate, brings about better body awareness and compassion.

The diaphragm is nestled at the bottom of the breastbone, underneath and behind the bottom six ribs, and separates the abdominal cavity from the chest cavity under the ribs. It is attached to the lumbar vertebrae, so it plays a key part in stabilizing the spine.

The obliques extend from the ribs to the iliac crest of the pelvis (the curved bone below your waist that forms part of your hip), and their main job is to support the abdomen against the pull of gravity and maintain the cavity. They also help with side bending.

Muscles on the back of the core include the quadratus lumborum (QL) and the erectors. The QL is used for side bending and stabilizes the side of the lumbar spine. When this muscle is tight, pain can be felt in the hip or glutes. The multifidius muscle also has an important stabilizing role.

The pelvic floor sits in a sling across the bottom and back of the pelvis. We tend to think of the need to strengthen and "draw up" the pelvic floor, but it is just as important to know how to intentionally relax the pelvic floor. A healthy pelvic floor will work with the diaphragm in moving with the breath.

The transverse abdominis is a very important deep muscle that goes from front to back, supporting the abdominal cavity and stabilizing the lumbar spine. It helps to maintain good posture and is used in strong exhalations, such as sneezing.

The rectus abdominis not only helps with reality-TV careers. It is used to stabilize the pelvis, and to fold forward when getting out of a chair. Weak muscle tone here can also contribute to lower-back pain. It is important to note that you can have a strong rectus abdominis that is not especially visible – having prominent 'abs' owes more to what you eat (or don't eat) and your genetics.

To "engage" the core, tense up, but don't pull in: it feels as though you are about to do a small cough. You'll notice that the front of the core will engage by about 30 per cent: no more or you start to put a "dent" in the core cylinder structure, throwing off its structural stability.

In a standing position, use the engagement of the legs, by connecting the feet to the ground, and trigger the engagement of the buttocks, hips, pelvis, back and torso muscles. When we add breathing to this, we can find a universal core engagement. The relation from the floor up to the core can provide a considerable degree of strength that simply working the "core muscles" themselves on their own will struggle to do.

Exercises for the Core

Dead Bug

This is a targeted move that engages
back and front core.

1. Lying on your back, raise either
alternate arms or legs, or both.

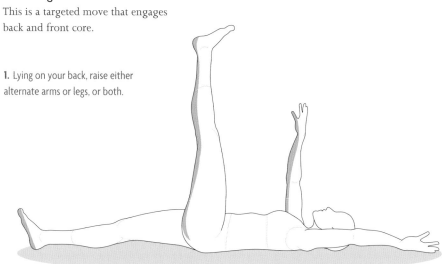

2. Keep the back in a neutral arch,
so that you can feel the back
muscles stabilize.

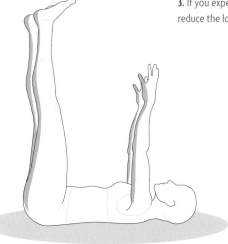

3. If you experience back pain,
reduce the load to the legs or arms.

Tiger Plank

This allows you to feel the "floor-to-core" relationship through your hands and feet and engage the side of the core, too.

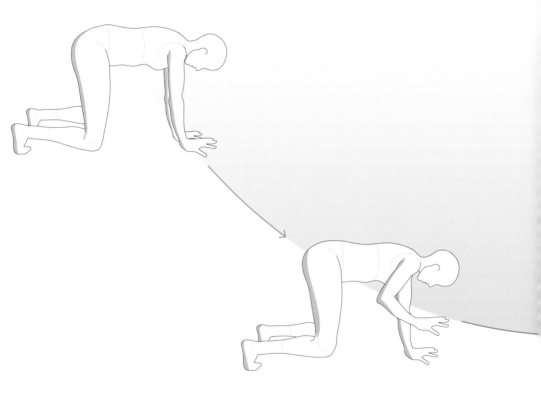

1. Start in All Fours (see page 138), with the toes tucked under. Push the toes down, engage the back and lift the knees so that they are hovering off the floor.

2. Use the outside edge and heel of the hands to engage the back and armpit muscles: these are connected to your spinal erectors, obliques and abdominals.

3. Push the toes down to engage the legs and glutes: these are also interconnected to the core.

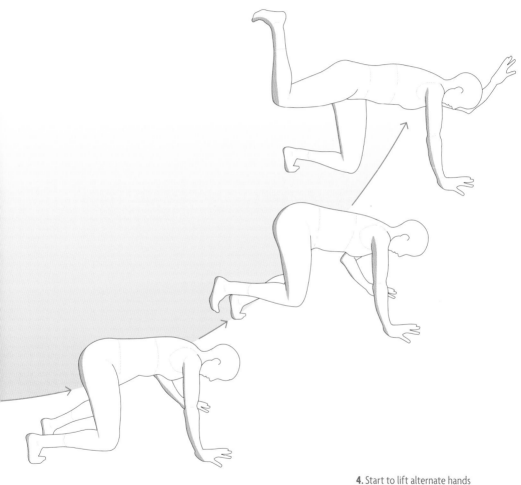

4. Start to lift alternate hands and toes (for example, left hand, right toes) – or even both! Bringing movement into the pose challenges the core even further.

Lunging Lasso

1. In a Lunge (see pages 104 and 107), keep the left hand by the hip: the right hand holds a "lasso".

2. Swing the lasso around your head: not just from your shoulder, but using the whole of your torso. Keep the front foot grounded and the leg engaged for stability.

3. Feel the trunk muscles engage as you move, to stop you from falling.

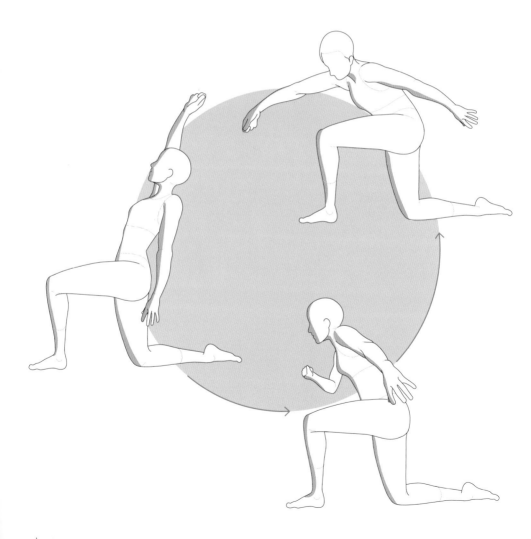

The Glutes

The "glutes" are the muscles in the buttocks and comprise the gluteus maximus ("glute max"), gluteus medius ("glute med") and gluteus minimus ("glute min"). They are instrumental in many common functional movements, such as walking, rising from sitting and balance.

The gluteus maximus is the largest muscle in the body, but all the glutes can become lazy. This is due to our sitting-based lifestyles, which doesn't encourage their use. When the glutes are not firing correctly, other muscles will take over their function, such as the hip flexors and lower back.

Gluteal weakness is often due to long periods of sitting on them, when they become over-stretched. Asymmetry at the pelvis can also affect them, as we weight-bear more favourably through our dominant leg and cause it to be stronger and more stable. And if you have injured any lower limb structure, the body inhibits the gluteals to slow you down.

Traditional yoga doesn't necessarily enhance the gluteal muscles and often can reinforce the front line of the body (see Muscle Chains, pages 38–41). This front line is often overworked already from sitting. Intentionally activating the glutes by keeping the knee slightly bent and pushing down through the heel will counteract this tendency.

Exercises for the Glutes

Prone Leg Extensions

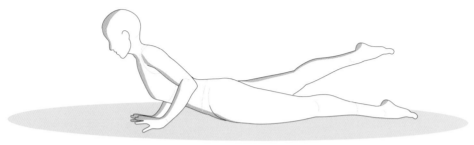

1. Lying face down, practise lifting each leg, keeping it straight. It doesn't matter how high it comes, as long as the pelvis stays level and touching the mat.

2. Notice the engagement of your hamstrings in the back of the leg, and of the glutes in your buttocks. If you feel this in your lower back, you can lower the head and chest to the floor instead.

M Wall-Sitting

Props: a block.

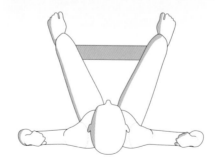

1. Lie down, with the feet wide and flat against the wall and knees bent: your legs will make an M shape in front of you.

2. Squeeze a block between the knees.

3. Lift one foot slowly away from the wall, without losing the squeeze on the block. Repeat with the other foot.

4. You might find that one foot comes up better than the other, or that one or both feet don't lift at all.

5. Notice the engagement in the side of your hip/buttocks: this is the gluteus medius.

Speed Skater

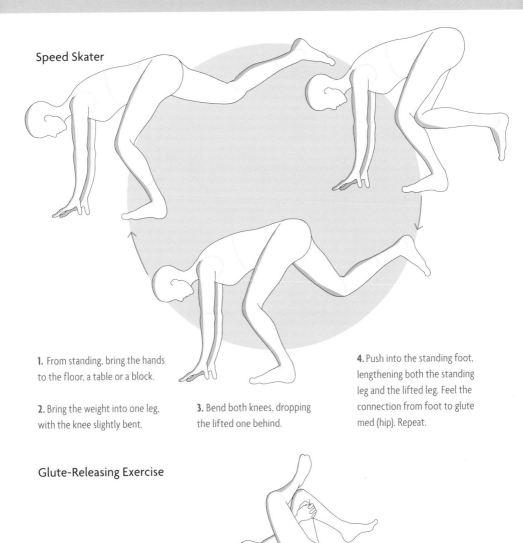

1. From standing, bring the hands to the floor, a table or a block.

2. Bring the weight into one leg, with the knee slightly bent.

3. Bend both knees, dropping the lifted one behind.

4. Push into the standing foot, lengthening both the standing leg and the lifted leg. Feel the connection from foot to glute med (hip). Repeat.

Glute-Releasing Exercise

1. Lying on the back, cross the thighs and hold the shins, ankles or feet. Rock a little.

2. Notice the sensation in the glute of the top thigh.

3. For a more knee-friendly release, try Sleeping Pigeon (see page 191).

The Hips

Our hips and pelvis are crucial in most everyday functional movement, including walking, bending down and balancing. The purpose of the hips is to keep us moving and they need to be stable and balanced.

The "hip" commonly refers to the insertion of the top of the femur (thigh) bone into the pelvis at the acetabulum; and then to 20 muscles, which are often small, around the joint, which helps it to move and stabilizes it. It may help to remember that the whole of our upper body rests on the top of the two thigh bones: the hips, pelvis, thighs and lower back have a very interconnected relationship.

Our hips are a ball-and-socket joint, which offers several ranges of movement: forward and back, side to side and rotation. When we sit, our hips are externally rotated, which causes stretching across the hips, buttocks and lower back.

Pelvic movement will affect the rest of the body, due to the pelvis's relationship with the spine and the thigh bones. Practising movement in the pelvis will free up other parts of the body, bringing mobility and relieving stiffness.

Sitting causes tightness in the hip flexors, and often the rest of the front body is tight, too. The hip flexors and lower back may be asked to do the work of the glutes when our bottoms get lazy, so they get tired. What often appears to be hip or back pain can be rectified by strengthening the glutes (see page 87).

Yoga poses – especially some of the more advanced ones – can put our hips into extreme ranges of motion that can damage the cartilaginous surfaces of the joint. This in turn can lead to irritation, possible inflammation and maybe even arthritis. To prevent this, moderation is key, in terms of the types of poses practised, their frequency, the range of motion used and whether stabilizing exercises are practised as well.

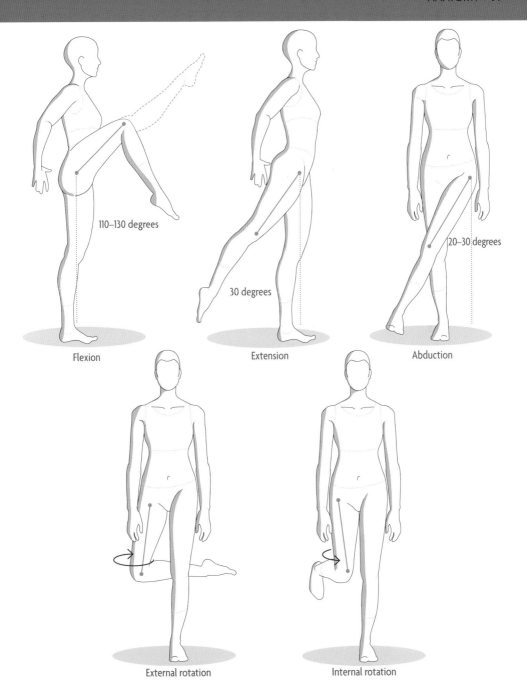

110–130 degrees

Flexion

30 degrees

Extension

20–30 degrees

Abduction

External rotation

Internal rotation

Exercises for the Hips

These sequences are designed to build stability and mobility through the hips, while also encouraging awareness of how pelvic movement influences the rest of the body. You can also explore the hips using the Active and Lounging Pigeon options on pages 188 and 189.

Rolling Lunge

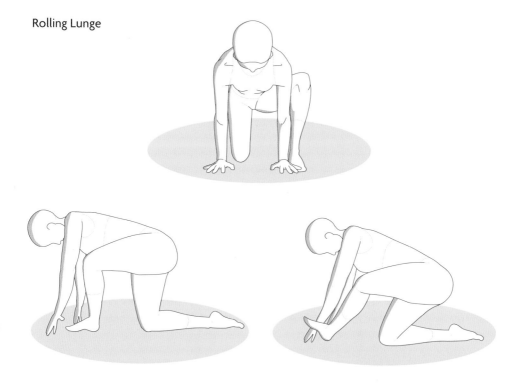

1. In Low Lunge (see page 104), with hands or fingertips on the floor or a block inside the front foot, start to shift your weight through the outside edge of the front foot.

2. Shift the weight through the toes, inside edge, heel and outside edge. Move slowly and go in both directions.

3. As you move, notice what is happening elsewhere in the body: the front thigh, the front hip, the back hip, the back leg. Notice how they respond to the simple shifting of weight through your foot.

Active Windscreen Wipers

1. Sitting with the knees bent and the feet wider than the hips (hands behind you), drop the knees from side to side, noticing the range of movement through the hips. Lean back as much as you need. Keep the feet wide.

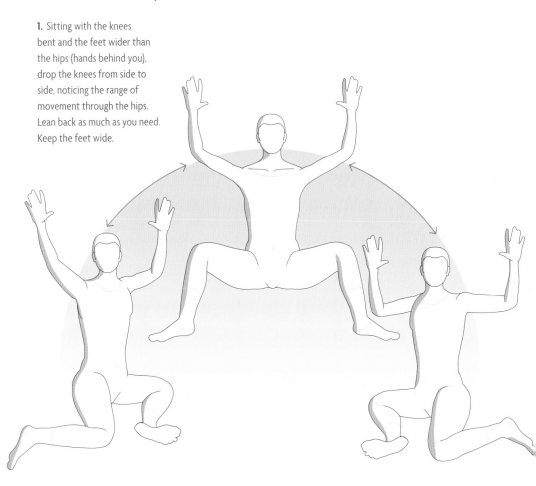

2. Notice how the hip can lift to facilitate a wider range of movement.

3. Practise taking alternate hands off the floor, and notice what engages through the body to keep you moving.

4. Practise it with both arms lifted: using the core, hip and leg strength to find an active movement.

The Legs and Feet

How our feet interact with the ground dictates our body's structure and response. The legs and feet support our entire body and take our weight whenever we stand, walk or run. Furthermore, if the foot-to-earth connection has imbalances, this will be reflected further up the legs, into the pelvis and above.

Feet and Ankles

The foot and ankle involve 26 small bones, 33 joints and more than 100 muscles, ligaments and tendons, all of which contribute to the essential dynamic movement of the foot. The intricate relationships between the lower leg and the foot indicate how a foot imbalance can affect the rest of the body. The sole of the foot is covered with nerve endings which send messages up the legs about muscle engagement and positioning.

When grounding the feet, we are looking for weight spread across the ball and outside edge of the foot and the heel, with the toes also engaged. This enables the main medial longitudinal arch of the foot to remain lifted and stabilizes the knees. When standing, you can put more weight in the heels or balls of the feet and observe the rest of your body responding to this shift.

Knees

The knee joint mediates the forces coming down from the hip and up from the foot, while permitting a considerable range of movement. If your knee hurts, it is most likely coming from the hip, ankle or foot, unless there is a direct trauma to the knee itself.

Other poses that affect the knee are standing poses, where the knee joint can be locked out. When the knee is locked out, considerable force is placed on the joint; when the knee is bent, the force is absorbed by the surrounding muscles. Poses that involve direct contact of the knee with the floor, such as All Fours (see page 138), can also cause issues, where the pressure on the floor can cause cartilage to wear away, leading to pain at the pressure point. Using a cushion or blanket to protect the knee is a good idea, even if you don't feel any pain at the moment.

Hamstrings

Hamstrings are designed for stability, as they help us to walk and run, so they are not intended to stretch very much. Stretching can feel good but if we overdo it, the muscle stops stretching, but the ligaments and tendons stretch instead, often pulling at insertion points in the buttocks and knee. For a different way to release the hamstrings, see the Lazy Tail Wag exercise opposite.

Exercise for the Legs and Feet

Lazy Tail Wag

Rather than stretching the hamstrings, we can massage them instead. You can also use foot pressure to stabilize the knee in Warrior 2 (see page 100).

1. In Low Lunge (see page 104), move the hips back so that the front leg lengthens and the back knee bends, with fingertips on the floor or hands on a block. Keep the front knee bent – this isn't about stretching.

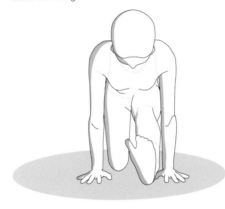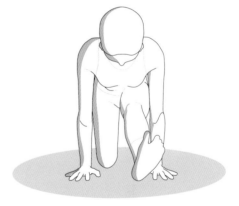

2. Slowly and lazily start to move your tailbone from side to side.

3. Allow – don't force – the hips, legs and front foot also to move from side to side. The front foot will pivot on the heel.

4. Notice the hamstrings in the back of the front leg moving and rubbing against each other, having a massage!

Poses

The following poses are described in the spirit of experimenting to move energy. Traditional versions of poses have been included, as well as ways to explore, modify and change them. In some cases a passive or restorative version is also included, for relaxation. In these poses you can set a timer to stay in them for a few minutes.

In a lot of yoga classes there is an emphasis on doing poses correctly. In this book, as long you as you are stable, have buoyancy and the freedom to breathe, then you are good to go. Yoga poses are tools for embodiment, so you are looking more at how they *feel*, rather than what they look like. As you practise it's important to learn how to notice what works, what is interesting and what is useful *for you*. If something hurts, don't do it! If something is unavailable to you, don't push it: use a block or a table; try a different version or move on to something else. Yoga practice is all about cultivating awareness in the body, not making perfect shapes.

The Change It Up! sections provide examples of how you can take a traditional *asana* and investigate different movement patterns, or ranges of motion, that can change your experience of the pose. When you come into a pose, negotiate with it. This might mean changing a foot or hand position so that you feel more stable; noticing where you are engaging or opening in the body or exploring different ways that you can move. After a few moments of this, find a comfortable or interesting place to pause for a few breaths, perhaps sending your breath into the spaces you have created. Then move on to a different version, the other side or a new pose, and repeat.

Ensure you breathe softly and steadily through the nose and pay attention to when the breath gets faster or catches, or if you're holding your breath. These are all signs that you are moving into a stress response and out of a relaxed state.

To practise, you'll need comfortable clothes; a mat or at least some cushioning for the knees and your bony bits; and blocks or any other props you might wish to use, including a chair or table, if needed. Put on some music and have a play!

Mountain Pose (*Tadasana*)

This pose is a wonderful way to find stillness and stability in the body. Mountain Pose is like a standing meditation: see if you can stand, relax and breathe. Mountain Pose is also the foundation of many standing poses, so practising distributing weight and engaging the feet here will help with other poses.

1. Stand upright with your arms by your side and your weight distributed equally through both legs.

2. Adjust the distance of the feet to find a place where the pelvis feels stable. Put more weight into the outside edge of the feet and heels, keeping the balls and toes in contact with the floor.

3. Soften the knees, so that the knee joints are not locked. If you notice your knees rolling in toward each other, put more weight into the outside edge of the foot. Close your eyes and shift your weight from foot to foot until you feel your pelvis is completely supported by your legs.

4. Bring attention to your torso. Are you puffing out your chest, rounding your shoulders or sticking out your buttocks? Gently move the spine until you feel equal space in front and behind the body. Allow the weight to drop into the feet and find your breath.

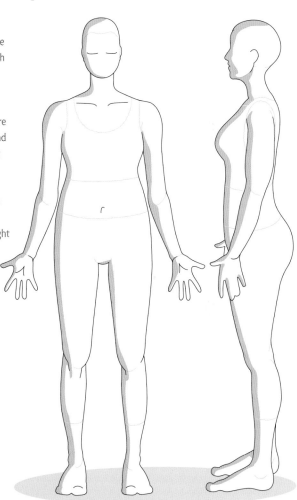

Forward Fold

Forward Folds bring us into relationship with the back line of our bodies (see page 39), and different variations can activate and open different parts of this muscle chain.

1. From standing, bend the knees as if you were going to sit down, and start to roll down the spine. Tuck in your chin, roll your shoulders forward and round through the back, until you get a slight hinge at the hips.

2. Keep the knee joints soft or bent.

3. Place the hands on the floor or on a block or chair, or just dangle them.

4. Shift your weight from foot to foot, and adjust the distance between the feet so it feels comfortable.

5. Put more weight into the outside edge of the feet and heels, keeping the balls and toes in contact with the floor.

6. Keep the knees bent and the tummy toward the thighs in this pose. The head should feel heavy.

7. Explore shifting your weight between the feet or making circles with the ankles.

8. To come out of the pose, roll up, keeping the chin tucked in and the hips moving over ankles until you're standing.

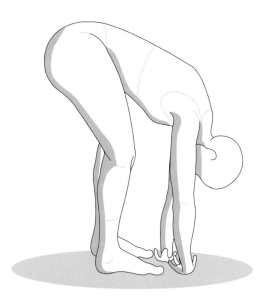

CHANGE IT UP!

▶ Half Lift

1. Alternatively, with the hands on the floor or on a block or chair, slowly lengthen the legs and then lift the chest.

2. Keep the back of the neck long, but find space across the collarbones.

3. Avoid locking out the knees.

4. Notice the lengthening of the back line of the body.

5. To come out, bend the knees and then fold over the thighs, back into the previous version of Forward Fold.

▶ Wide-Legged Forward Fold

1. Find a wide-leg standing position that feels stable, so you can connect the feet to the floor and there is some tension between the legs. Bend the knees, drop the pelvis behind you and slowly bring the hands to the floor or on a block or chair.

2. Adjust the foot position until you are balanced and stable, so that the thigh bones are not jamming into the pelvis and the feet aren't too far apart. You can shift your weight from foot to foot, or slowly lengthen through the back of the legs until they are straight. Notice the difference in the range of movement in this wide-legged fold.

3. To come out, bend the knees, drop the pelvis, lift the chest and then drive through the feet to stand up.

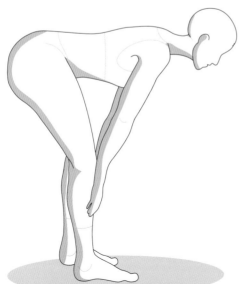

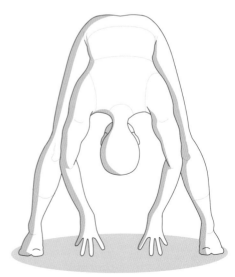

Warrior 2 (*Virabhadrasana* II)

There are several Warrior poses, and Warrior 2 and
3 are included in this book. Warrior 1 is omitted,
as it can place stress on the back knee and lower
back: use High Lunge (see page 107) instead.

1. From Mountain Pose (see page 97), step back with
your left foot and turn the heel down and toes out,
so that the foot is flat.

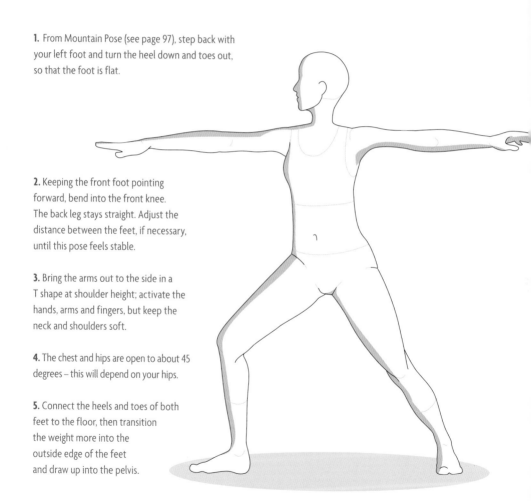

2. Keeping the front foot pointing
forward, bend into the front knee.
The back leg stays straight. Adjust the
distance between the feet, if necessary,
until this pose feels stable.

3. Bring the arms out to the side in a
T shape at shoulder height; activate the
hands, arms and fingers, but keep the
neck and shoulders soft.

4. The chest and hips are open to about 45
degrees – this will depend on your hips.

5. Connect the heels and toes of both
feet to the floor, then transition
the weight more into the
outside edge of the feet
and draw up into the pelvis.

CHANGE IT UP!

▶ Explore Range of Motion

1. In Warrior 2, explore your range of motion by moving the front arm in circles, as well as noticing the impact of the arm movement on the rest of the body.

2. Stay mindful of the hips and knees as you do this.

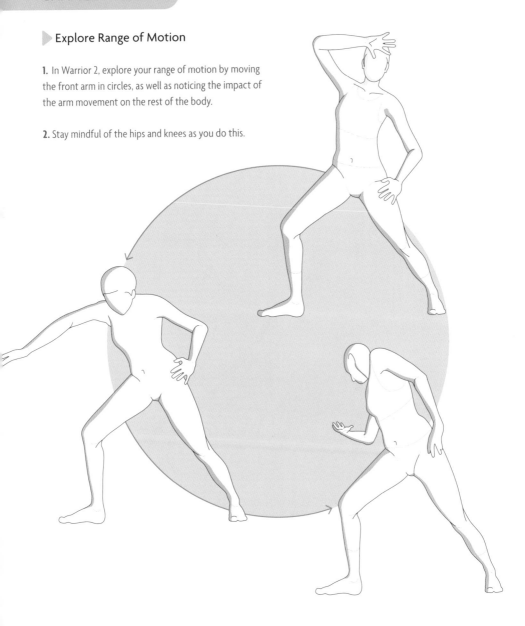

▶ **Transition to Reverse Warrior**

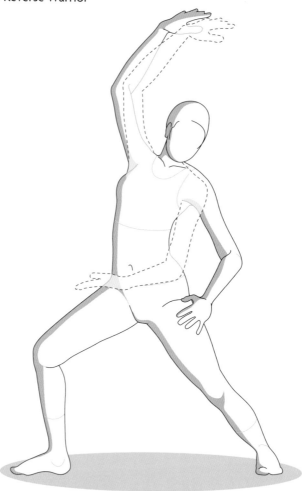

1. From Warrior 2, lift the front arm, lean back a little.

2. Take the back hand down the back of the thigh, or onto the lower back.

3. Notice the opening of the front and side torso.

▶ Transition to Rainbow Warrior

1. From Reverse Warrior, reach forward with the lifted arm and place the hand or forearm on the front knee.

2. Extend the back arm toward the sky or over the top ear.

3. Notice the space along the top side of the body and the engagement in the legs and trunk for support.

4. Move between Rainbow Warrior and Reverse Warrior.

5. You can also play with the arm positions: pointing the back arm forward in Reverse Warrior, and the front arm backward in Rainbow.

6. Make sure you are stable through your feet and front knee especially.

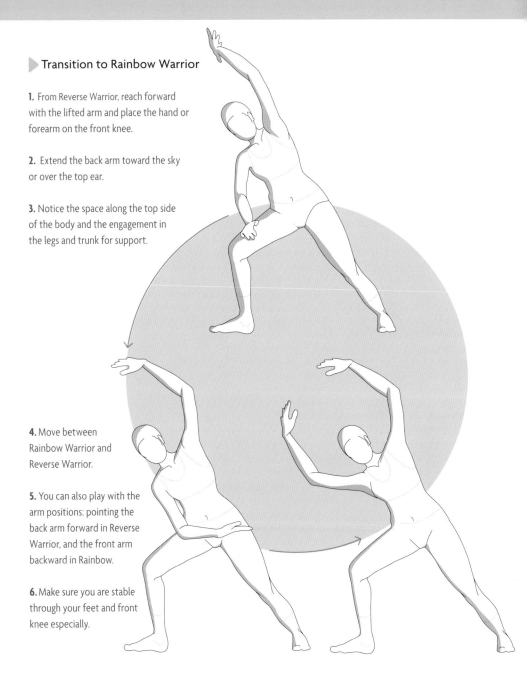

Low Lunge *(Anjaneyasana)*

Lunges are great for mobilizing and strengthening the hips and legs.

1. From hands and knees, step the right foot forward, just to the outside of your right hand.

2. Shift the weight into the outside edge and heel of the front foot, while keeping the toes connected to the floor. The hands can stay down on the floor or a block.

3. Push through the foot and lift the chest into a vertical position. You can use your hands against your thigh to assist you, if needed.

4. The front foot should be in a position where you can push firmly straight down through the heel into the floor, supporting the knee. The back foot supports the pelvis.

5. Bring the arms up alongside the ears, keeping the shoulders and neck relaxed.

6. Lengthen through the sides of the torso, ensuring the shoulders don't come up by the ears.

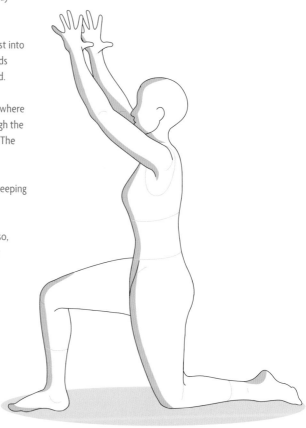

CHANGE IT UP!

▶ Twisted Lunge (*Parivrtta Anjaneyasana*)

1. From a Low Lunge with the left foot forward, bring the right hand down to the floor or on a block, where it will support the body.

2. Turn the torso toward the bent front leg.

3. You are looking for length in the spine and no stress in the back of the neck and skull.

4. Perhaps take the front foot wider and turn it out, so you can explore movement with the top arm.

5. Bring the right elbow and forearm to the floor or a block. Pay attention to the inside of the left leg: it should not be too strong here.

6. Ensure your body weight is supported, that there is integration from the supporting hand or forearm into the right side of the body, then lift the back knee.

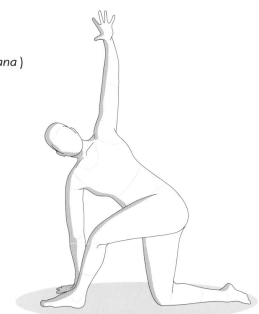

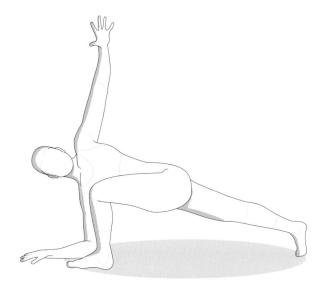

▶ Low-Lunging Cow/Cat

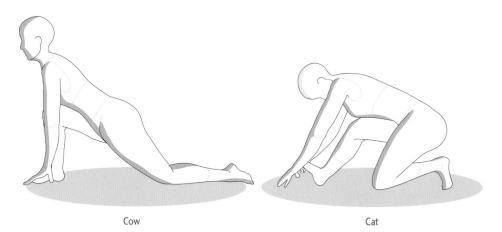

Cow   Cat

1. From a Low Lunge, lift the chest, with elbows into the side body, move the hips back and bend the front knee a little more: Cow.

2. Move the hips back, round the back and tuck the chin in; arms reach forward; front leg can lengthen: Cat.

3. Use the front foot to control the movement. Notice how all the joints from ankle to neck need to articulate to enable you to move in this way.

▶ Elastic Lunge

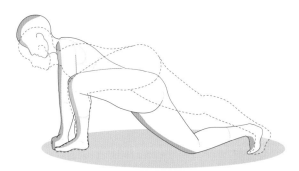

1. From a Low Lunge, lift the back knee, but keep it soft.

2. Shift the weight from front to back foot, allowing the knees to bend and the back leg to lengthen as you move.

3. Look to remain pliable as you shift the weight, rather than stretching deeply.

High Lunge (*Ashta Chandrasana*)

Lunges come in several variations to suit different people and situations, and this is a variation on the theme.

1. In a Low Lunge (see page 104), bring your hands to the floor and bring the front foot slightly more centrally between the hands. Tuck the back toes under.

2. Shift the weight between the feet, so that your pelvis feels suspended between the legs, then push through both feet to come up. You can use your hands on your thigh. Keep the weight in the big toe, outside edge and heel of the front foot.

3. Once the chest is lifted, you can reposition your back foot so you feel more stable. Try bringing it closer to the front or taking it wider, if you feel wobbly.

4. The back foot is balanced on the ball and toes, with the heel lifted. Keep the back knee bent or soft: there should be a sense of lightness in the pose.

5. The arms can come up by the ears, with the neck and shoulders staying soft.

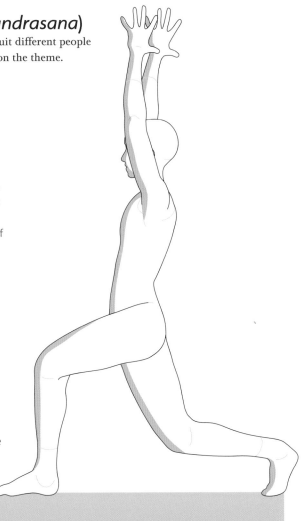

HOW TO MODIFY

- If coming into High Lunge is difficult, stay in Low Lunge.
- If the sensation in the hips is too strong, shorten the distance between the back and front knees/legs.
- If the back knee is uncomfortable on the floor, use a blanket for cushioning.
- If there is back pain, keep more of a bend in the back knee.

CHANGE IT UP!

Lunging Lasso

1. Practise your Lunging Lasso (see page 86) in a High Lunge. Remember to stay pliable in the pose and to move with the lasso!

Twist and Spiral

1. From a High Lunge with the left foot forward, bring the right elbow across the front thigh, as if you were carrying a plate in that hand; round the shoulders a little and tuck in the chin.

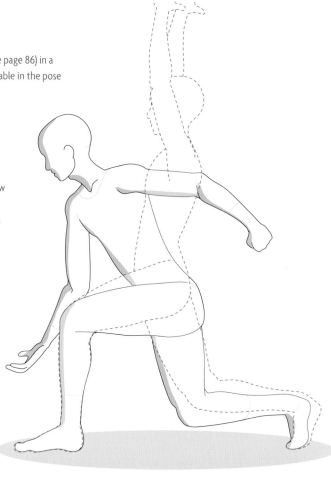

2. The elbow shouldn't touch the thigh: hover it and push down through the feet, engage the core and back, so you are stable in this position.

3. To come out, push off the front foot to help lift the torso and un-spiral.

4. Practising moving in and out of this twist is good for mobility and stability.

Winged Lunge

1. From a High Lunge, hinge from the hips and swing the arms back behind you like aeroplane wings.

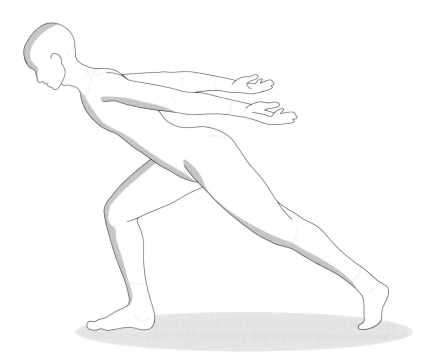

2. Notice the engagement of the back muscles to support the torso, as well as the front of the core.

3. Stay firm through the feet and glutes, to find that integrated support from the floor through the centre of the body.

4. You can move between Winged Lunge and High Lunge, or even Surfer (see page 127), to practise shifting weight and balance.

▶ Bend and Lengthen

1. In High Lunge, bend both knees as much as you can, with lifted arms.

2. Straighten both legs, without locking out the knee joints.

3. Bring the elbows down into the side ribs and imagine you are holding really heavy plates: feel the mid-back engage.

4. Move between the stances, paying attention to what needs to work and what lengthens.

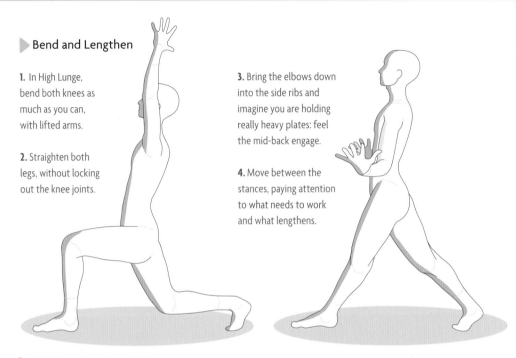

▶ High-Lunging Cow/Cat

1. As for Low-Lunging Cow/Cat (see page 106), except, for Cow the front knee bends and the back leg lengthens.

2. For Cat, the front leg lengthens and the back knee bends: this can feel strange – take it slowly!

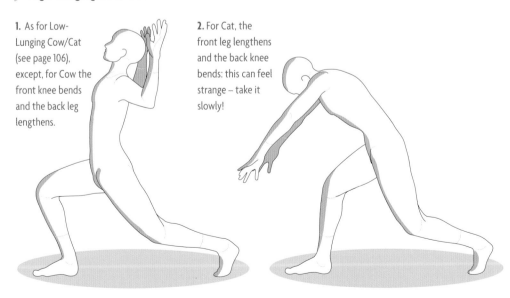

Tree Pose (*Vrksasana*)

Tree Pose is great for practising balance, especially when movement is added.

1. From standing, shift your weight into the right leg and soften the knee.

2. Bring up your left foot against the calf or thigh.

3. Where you put the foot will depend on the range of movement in your hip.

4. Keep the hips facing forward and the standing knee soft.

5. Find a focal point to rest your gaze on, to help your stability.

6. Bring the hands into the prayer position in front of the chest.

7. If you feel stable, you can bring the arms up alongside your ears.

8. Use a hand against a wall or table for support, if necessary.

9. Feel the foot-to-hip connection, supporting your weight.

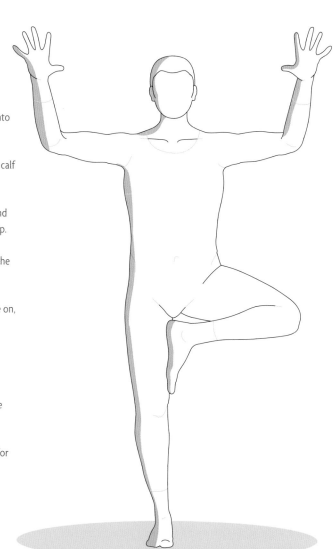

CHANGE IT UP!

▶ Twisted Tree

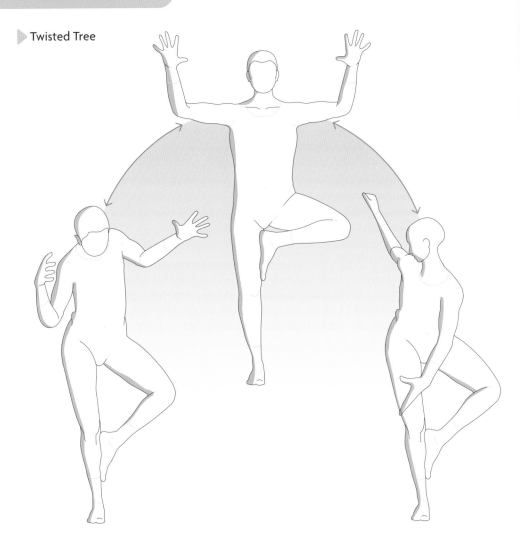

1. In Tree Pose, slowly bend the standing knee, to facilitate movement.

2. Move slowly – the arms, gentle twists – just finding new shapes.

3. Don't worry if you fall out of the position!

Angry Animal

1. In Tree Pose, take the lifted foot away from the inside of the standing leg and point the sole of the foot forward.

2. Bend the standing knee and allow the hips to move backward as if sitting on a chair. You may want to have the arms out to the side, for balance.

3. Look for what is happening through the hips to balance and extend the lifted leg. An angry face is optional!

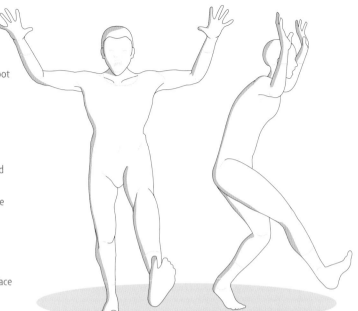

Standing Pigeon (*Kapotasana*)

1. In Tree Pose, bring the lifted ankle onto the standing knee.

2. Move the sit bones back a little, as the arms go alongside the head or come into the prayer position.

3. Notice the space created in the lifted hip, and the work happening in the supporting hip.

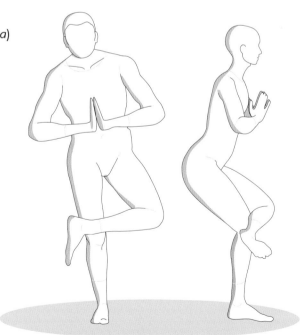

Warrior 3 and Half Moon Pose

These single-leg balances really fire up the glutes and hips.
Focus on how the foot is working to support the standing leg.

Warrior 3 (*Virabhadrasana* III)

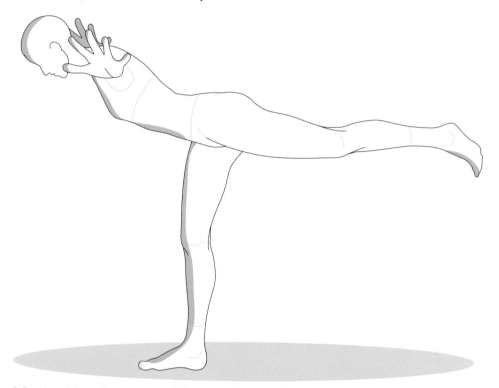

1. From Mountain Pose (see page 97), shift the weight into the right foot, bend the knee and hinge forward at the hips, lifting the left leg behind.

2. Keep the supporting knee bent, and the spine and back of the neck long.

3. Focus on the hamstrings lifting the back leg; you can also flex the toes to activate the foot more, which keeps the leg alive and working.

4. Notice the glutes and hips working in both legs: you may feel it most in the side of the hips.

5. Arms can be alongside you, like wings, for balance, or out to the side or alongside the ears.

6. Integrate across the shoulder blades, keeping the tops of the shoulders away from the ears, and the back muscles engaged, to stop the chest dipping.

HOW TO MODIFY

Hands can be placed on a wall, block, chair or table for support: ensure there is enough distance, so that the spine stays long.

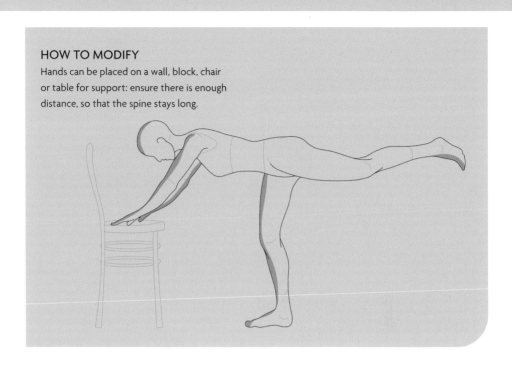

CHANGE IT UP!

▶ Standing Splits

1. In Warrior 3, bring the hands to the floor or onto blocks.

2. Push into the standing foot as you lengthen the standing leg.

3. Start to lift the back leg even higher as your nose comes toward your supporting knee.

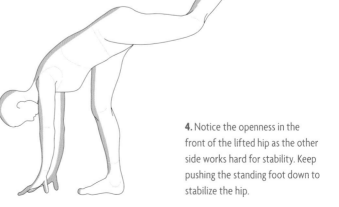

4. Notice the openness in the front of the lifted hip as the other side works hard for stability. Keep pushing the standing foot down to stabilize the hip.

Half Moon Pose (*Ardha Chandrasana*)

As with Warrior 3 (see page 114), focus on how the foot is working to support the standing leg.

HOW TO MODIFY

- The bottom hand can be placed on the floor or on a block or chair, if needed.
- This whole pose can be done against the wall: lean into the wall and use it for balance and support.

1. In Warrior 2 (see page 100), notice how the front knee is bent and the hips and torso are open to 45 degrees or so. Aim to keep this shape as you shift more weight into the front foot. You may want to shift between the back and front foot until you feel confident taking the weight into the front.

2. As the weight comes forward, the right hand points down to the ground.

3. Keeping the front knee bent and the body slightly open, bring your weight into the front foot and float the back leg up behind you.

4. The front knee should stay slightly bent to enable the glutes and leg muscles to take the weight of the body.

5. You can practise opening the hips a little more or extending the back leg, but aim to keep a sense of buoyancy in the pose.

CHANGE IT UP!

▶ Half Moon Bow (*Ardha Chandra Chapasana*)

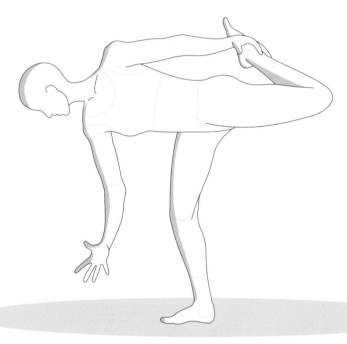

1. In Half Moon Pose, bend the lifted leg and reach for the foot with the lifted hand.

2. Move slowly to grasp the foot with the lifted hand, and take time for the weight to shift back through the supporting leg. Kick the foot into the holding hand to activate the leg.

3. Keep the standing knee bent, to ensure the foot and hip are working to support you.

Triangle

The aim of Triangle is to lengthen the inside of the legs and engage the side body. Some practitioners may find the modifications more comfortable, while more experienced yogis may find the other options interesting to explore.

Traditional Triangle (*Trikonasana*)

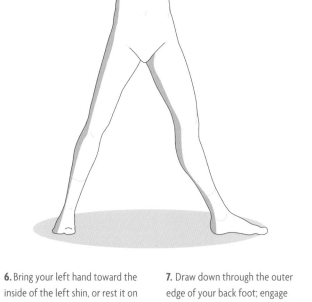

1. From Warrior 2 (see page 100), with the right leg back, straighten both legs without locking out the knees.

2. Raise your arms horizontally and activate the fingers.

3. Stabilize through the feet, finding the outside edges, heels and big toes.

4. Reach through your front hand in the same direction as your front foot is pointed. As the weight moves over the front leg, put more weight in the back foot; you may feel the right hip move slightly away from the left hand.

5. Fold at the left hip, keeping the spine long. Engage through the side body to keep the torso from dropping downward.

6. Bring your left hand toward the inside of the left shin, or rest it on the floor or a block, and slowly open through the torso toward the left.

7. Draw down through the outer edge of your back foot; engage across the back body, to integrate the shoulder blades and muscles of the mid-back.

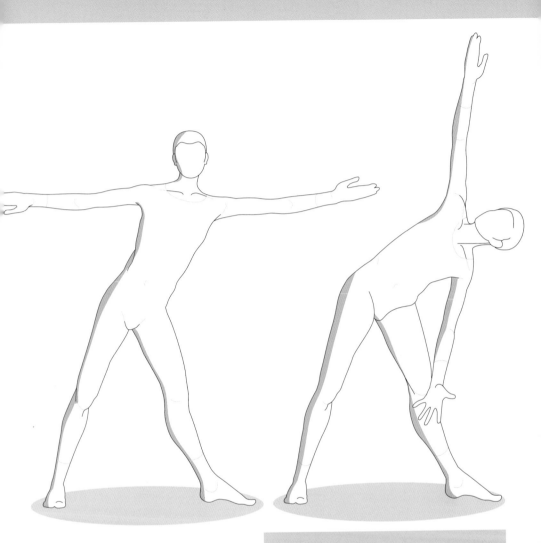

8. To come out, bend the front knee, push through the foot and slowly lift the torso.

HOW TO MODIFY

- The supporting hand is on the thigh and the torso pointing slightly upward. This opens the legs, with less pressure through the hips.
- Instead of a block, you could use a chair for the supporting hand.

CHANGE IT UP!

▶ Vanda's Triangle

An alternative to Traditional Triangle proposed by renowned yoga teacher Vanda Scaravelli was to stand with the feet much closer together.

1. From a standing position, step the right foot back, so the toes are about 2.5cm (1in) behind the heel of the front foot, but a comfortable distance apart width-wise.

2. Adjust the feet so that both sets of toes point forward. Find stability through the feet: spread the toes, plant the heels.

3. Keeping the legs straight, but not locking either knee, hinge forward at the hips, with the torso parallel to the ground. The hands can come onto blocks, a chair or the floor.

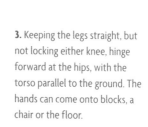

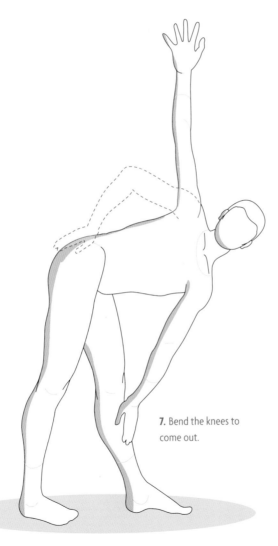

4. Reach your right hand behind you and feel for the back of the pelvis.

5. Keep the hand on the pelvis and start to twist through the bottom of the ribcage and mid-back. Use the right hand to check the pelvis is level as you twist: the twist is through the thoracic.

6. The right arm can extend to the ceiling, but make sure the back of the pelvis stays level.

7. Bend the knees to come out.

▶ Reverse Triangle (*Viparita Trikonasana*)

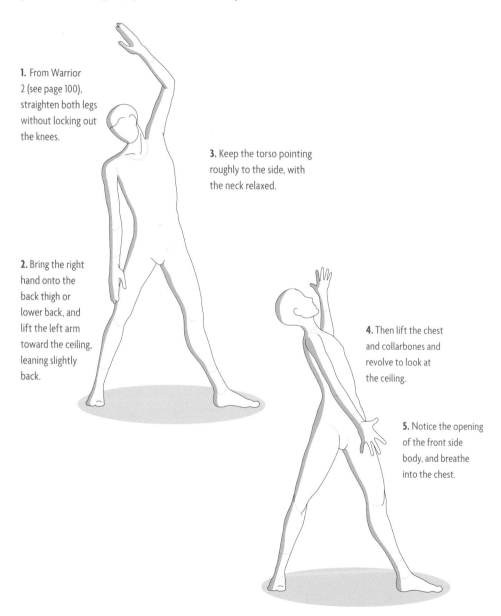

1. From Warrior 2 (see page 100), straighten both legs without locking out the knees.

3. Keep the torso pointing roughly to the side, with the neck relaxed.

2. Bring the right hand onto the back thigh or lower back, and lift the left arm toward the ceiling, leaning slightly back.

4. Then lift the chest and collarbones and revolve to look at the ceiling.

5. Notice the opening of the front side body, and breathe into the chest.

Horse Pose (*Vatayanasana*)

This is a fun, strong, dynamic pose that works the legs.

1. Stand with the feet a comfortable distance apart, so that it feels as though your body is well supported.

2. Turn your feet out and bend into your knees, without sticking out your buttocks too much.

3. You can stay in this squat position by engaging the outer edges of the feet, heels and toes and drawing the inner thighs together. Stand up when you need to!

4. Engage with the feet-to-hip connection.

5. Alternatively, with the knees bent, you can shift your weight from foot to foot, moving the hips as you do so.

6. Or you can move between straight legs and the squat position.

7. The arms can be in the prayer position, out to the side or overhead.

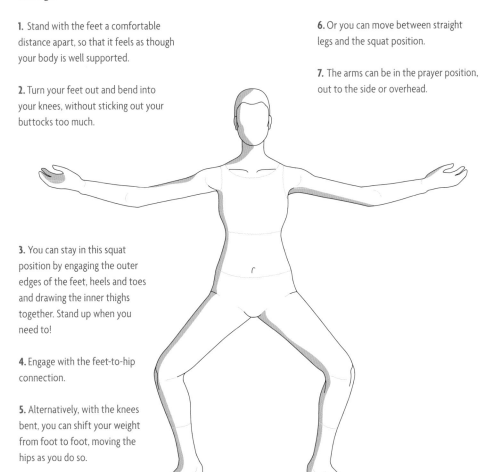

▶ Add Eagle Arms (*Garudasana*)

This is wonderful for opening across the back, and feeling the connection from the back into the legs.

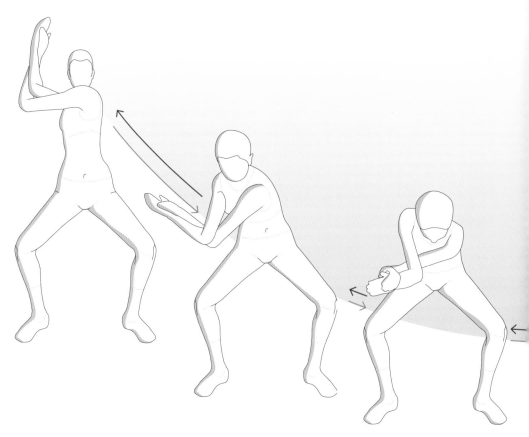

1. In Horse Pose, find Eagle Arms (see page 180) and turn the head from side to side.

2. Start with small circles of the elbows in both directions.

3. Make the circles bigger, by bending the knees then dropping the elbows toward one knee, across the floor and up again.

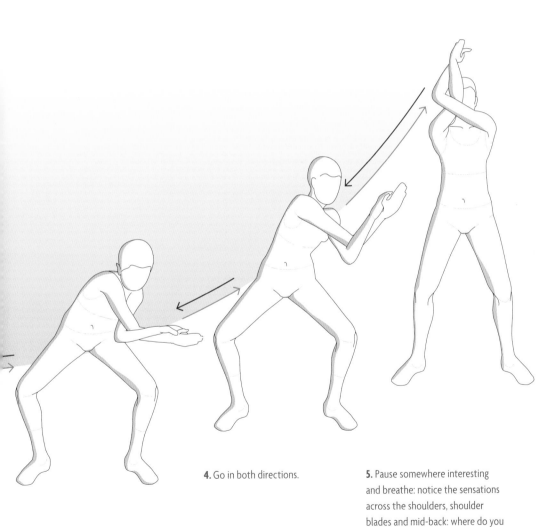

4. Go in both directions.

5. Pause somewhere interesting and breathe: notice the sensations across the shoulders, shoulder blades and mid-back: where do you want to breathe into?

▶ Step into Standing Curtsey

This is great for practising shifting your weight and balance, as well as opening up the side body.

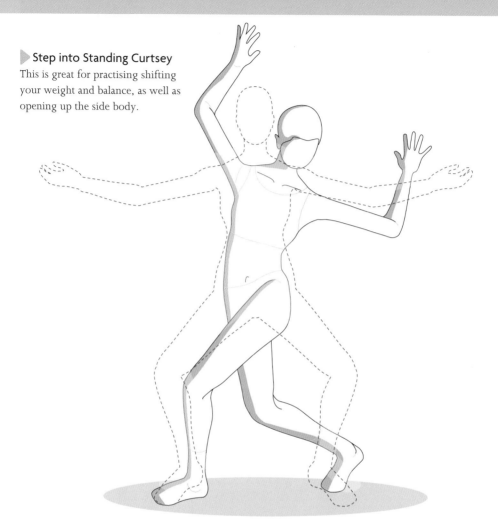

1. From Horse Pose, push off the right foot and step it behind the left foot, balancing on the ball of the right foot.

2. Bend both knees: you might need to adjust the placement of the back foot so that the knees bend comfortably.

3. Take the arms up alongside the ears, and keep the neck soft, with the gaze down to the left a little.

4. Breathe into where the spiral shape has created space in the side and back of the body.

5. To come out, push off the ball of the right foot and step back to Horse Pose.

6. You can practise moving between the two poses, and even add Eagle Arms (see page 124) by bringing the right arm over the left in Standing Curtsey.

▶ Surfer

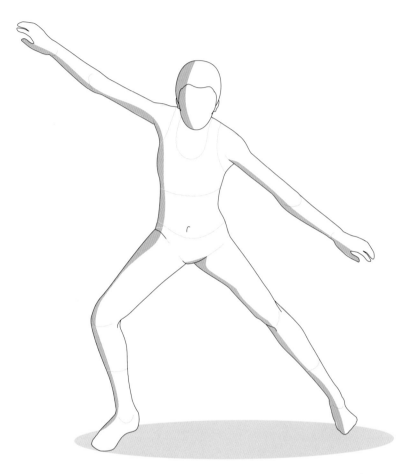

1. From Horse Pose, turn the toes in a little.

2. Bend one knee and lengthen the other leg; extend the arms away, reaching one hand toward the foot of the straight leg and the other hand upward.

3. The spine is long, the back of the neck relaxed.

4. Pulse through the foot of the bent knee to fire up the glutes and hamstrings. This is Surfer.

5. Shift the weight from side to side to make the pose more dynamic.

6. You can also twist toward the bent knee.

Chair and Squats

These are all variations on a squat, and can be difficult if your bone structure does not allow it. Always adjust your feet and ensure that the knees are happy.

Chair Pose (*Utkatasana*)

1. Standing, move the pelvis backward as your knees bend; keep the chest lifted.

2. Allow the arms to come up by the ears.

3. You may need to adjust the position of the feet, perhaps taking them a little wider, to allow for the rotation of the hip joint.

4. If having the arms by the ears feels tight in the shoulders, keep the arms straight, but take them further away from the ears.

5. Feel the muscles across the mid-back and under the armpit engage, as well as the glutes and legs.

6. Bring the tummy onto the thighs and move into a Forward Fold (see page 98), or push through the feet to stand, keeping the spine long.

7. You can also take Chair Pose into Standing Pigeon (see page 113) or High Lunge (see page 107).

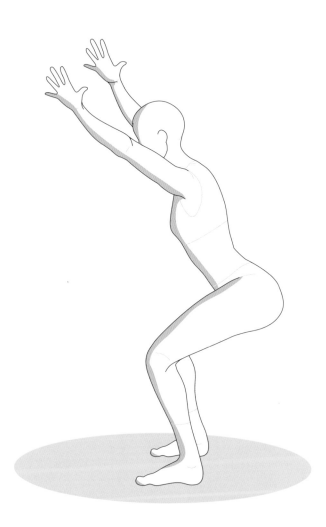

CHANGE IT UP!

▶ Hunchback

1. From Chair Pose, allow the pelvis to move forward, the tailbone to drop and the back to round.

2. The shoulders will round and the chin tuck in; the arms point forward, creating space across the back.

3. You can return to Chair Pose by lifting the chest and allowing the pelvis to move back. This is like a standing Cow/Cat!

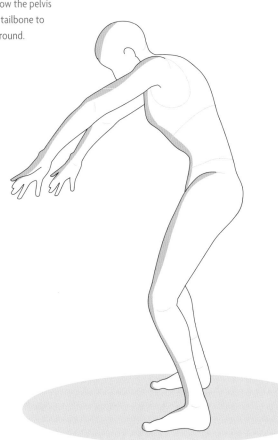

Squat (*Malasana*)

In a squat, the pelvis drops behind the knees.
For those with knee problems, take the pelvis
level with the knees, with the feet wider.

1. From Forward Fold (see page
98), bring the hands to the floor
and lift the heels. Slowly lower
your pelvis toward the heels as you
bend the knees.

2. Take the feet wider to
accommodate the hips; the
feet and knees can point out or
forward. Practise your balance.

3. The hands can stay
on the floor or in the
prayer position.

4. This is a strong
external hip rotation:
pay attention to the
feeling in the hips,
lower back and knees.

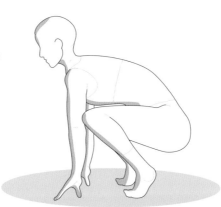

HOW TO MODIFY

- You can place your hands on a block, chair
  or table for balance.

- You can place a block underneath the heels,
  so that the weight can move out of the balls
  of the feet: be careful to remain engaged
  through the legs and hips and not go into the
  end-range of motion.

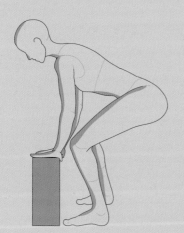

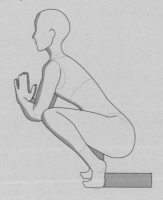

CHANGE IT UP!

▶ Half Squat

1. In Squat, turn the feet, knees and the whole body to the left until the left heel comes to the ground. Stay there and notice how this feels through the left hip.

2. Then swivel to the right and pause on this side.

3. Go from side to side, perhaps with the hands off the floor. You can also add a twist.

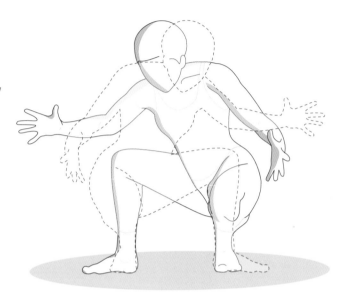

▶ Toe Squat

1. From kneeling, lift the buttocks so you can tuck all your toes under: make sure this includes the baby toes.

2. Place the hands on the floor under the shoulders. Gradually move the weight back into the toes by walking your hands in toward you. Maybe lift one and then both hands off the floor, bringing more weight into the pelvis.

3. With hands off the floor, can you bring the pelvis over the heels and sit with a tall spine?

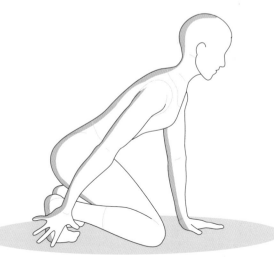

Planks

Planks are great for building integrated strength throughout the body.

Main Plank (*Phalakasana*)

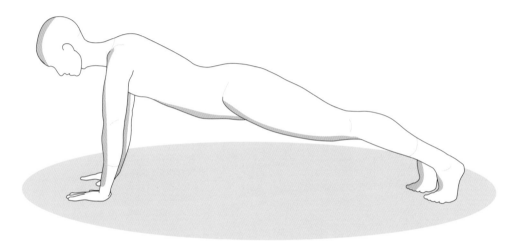

1. In All Fours (see page 138), position the hands where they support the shoulders.

2. Pay attention to the integration of the shoulder blades across the back, the muscles underneath them, and those under the armpits at the side body.

3. Slightly pull the hands toward each other and push down: this will prevent the chest collapsing. Keep the elbows slightly bent.

4. Keep this position and step one foot back, with the toes tucked under, then the other foot.

5. Look forward a little, so that the head doesn't drop.

6. Push through the heels and stay pliable – find subtle shifts and movements, adjusting the weight through the hands and feet.

7. Make some hip circles in both directions, or lift alternate hands and feet to make the pose more dynamic.

8. Knees can be on the ground, but keep the spine, including the back of the neck, long and the toes tucked under.

Forearm Plank

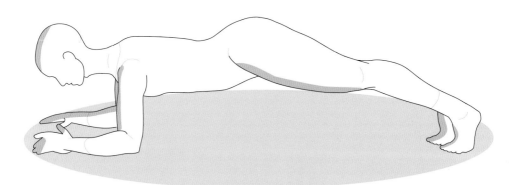

1. As for Main Plank (see opposite), but position the forearms under the shoulders.

2. Push the fingers, palms and arms into the ground to create strength and protraction in the shoulder blades.

3. Push back through the heels to create engagement throughout the whole body.

4. Avoid if you have rotator-cuff issues, as this pose is strong on the muscles around the armpits.

Side Plank A (*Parighasana*)

1. In All Fours (see page 138), take one leg back and ground the foot.

2. Spin the other ankle backward so that you face the side.

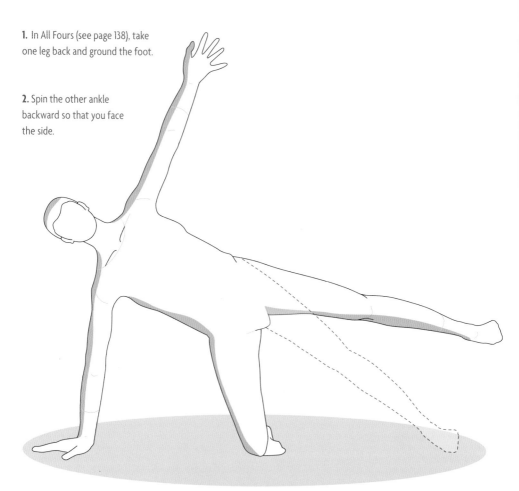

3. Lift the chest, opening to the side.

4. Keep the supporting elbow slightly bent, and find that integration around the armpit and shoulder blade.

5. Drive the supporting shin down into the floor for stability.

6. Explore movement with the top arm, noticing the connection into the side body, back and chest.

7. You can lift the extended leg up to hip height, to fire up the glutes and hips.

Side Plank B

1. In Low Lunge (see page 104), step the front foot so that it points to the side of the mat.

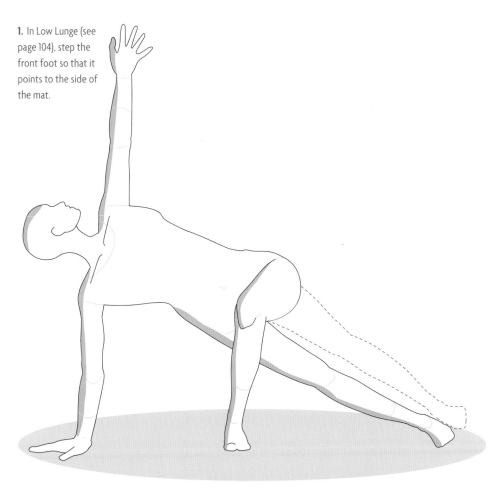

2. Support the opposite shoulder, lift the other knee and come onto the outside edge of that foot.

3. Lift the non-supporting hand.

4. Lower the hips and round the back. Then push with the feet, lift the hips and open to the ceiling.

5. Repeat two to three times; notice the strong foot-to-hip connection, and the engagement and opening of the sides of the body as you lift up.

Full Side Plank (*Vasisthasana*)

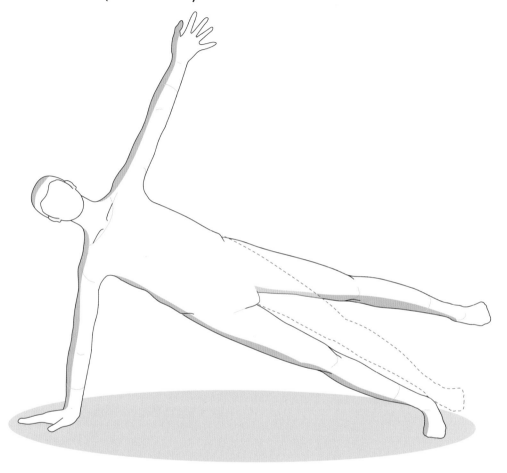

1. In Side Plank A (see page 134), lift the supporting knee, and extend this leg so it is underneath the other, with the feet either stacked or one behind the other. Engage the edges of the feet into the floor.

2. The support of the armpit, side body and mid-back must be engaged for this pose to be comfortable.

3. The top leg can also lift.

Tiger Plank

1. In All Fours (see page 138), tuck the toes under and find some pliability by bending the elbows, pushing into the heels and allowing the pelvis and spine to follow.

2. Lift alternate hands and then feet away from the floor.

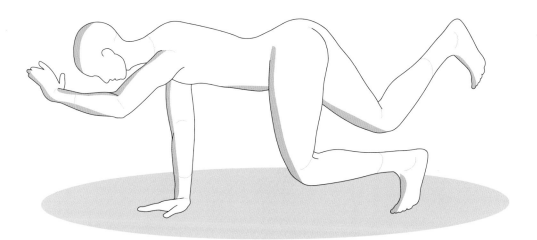

3. Let the body move and sway to accommodate the shift in weight.

4. Push through the heels to hover the knees off the floor: start to shift the weight from foot to foot and hand to hand, as you did in step 2.

5. If you are feeling okay, go ahead and lift alternate hands, feet – and even both. Let the body move!

6. Notice the weight shifting and the total body integration through the core as you move.

All Fours (*Bharmanasana*)

All Fours is an integral part of many poses. It can be hard on the wrists, so take rest when needed. You can also rotate the wrists like a flamenco dancer or pump your fingers into a fist for release.

1. Kneeling on all fours, bring your hands under your shoulders and your knees under your hips. Adjust the weight between your hands and knees until you feel the weight of your body is fully supported.

2. Soften but don't bend the elbows; take more weight into the little-finger side and heel of the hands, with all the fingers and thumbs connecting to the floor.

3. Tuck the toes under and notice any difference to your stability through the pelvis.

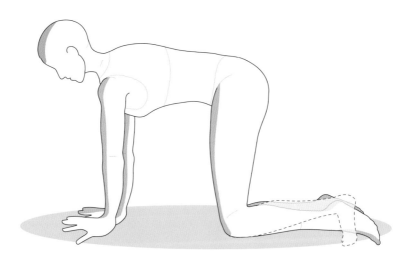

CHANGE IT UP!

▶ All Fours Hip, Rib and Shoulder Circles

1. In All Fours, make hip, rib and shoulder circles in both directions; can you create a figure eight? Play with the positions of the hands: wider, narrower, asymmetric: can you still make circles with the body? What do you notice in the torso as you change position?

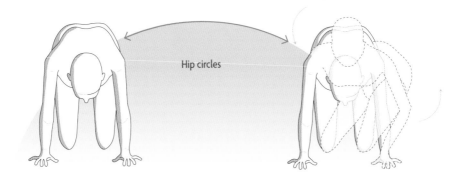

Hip circles

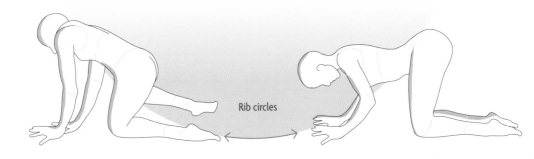

Rib circles

▷ All Fours Chest Opener (*Anahatasana*)

1. In All Fours, take the hands further
forward, keeping the hips over the
knees, and bring the head to the floor
or a block.

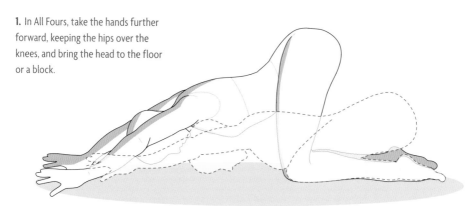

▷ All Fours Curtsey

1. In All Fours, take the left leg behind
the other and tuck the toes, as if doing a
curtsey. Push in and out of the toes; and
you can walk your hands further round
to the right to open up the side body.

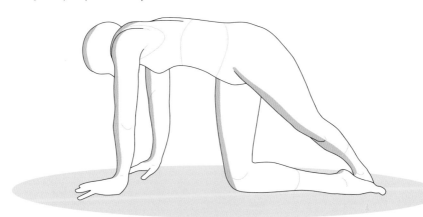

In the variations on pages 141–144, make sure the
hand on the floor is supporting the shoulder and
that the muscles around the armpit are engaged, by
finding the outside edge/little-finger side of the
hand. The toes are tucked under, for greater stability.

▶ Circle-Arm All Fours

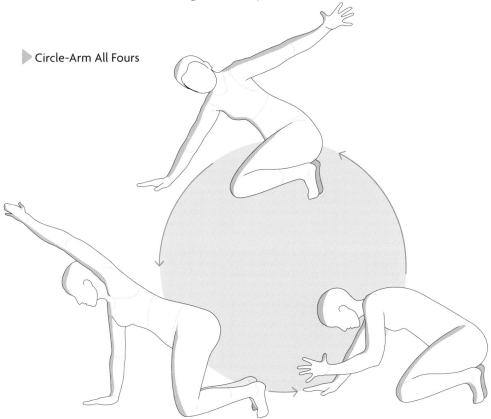

1. In All Fours, lift the left arm,
pointing the fingers forward. Take
the arm back past the ear behind
you, opening the chest. Allow the
hips to move back toward the heels.

2. Let the arm continue its circle,
from the legs along the floor and
back up toward the head. The hips
will lift back over the knees again.

3. Continue making arm circles,
going in each direction a few
times. Pay attention to the
connection between the hips,
torso and lifted arm.

Thread the Needle and Scoops

1. In All Fours, lift the right arm to the ceiling, allowing the chest to open.

2. Dive that hand under the supporting arm, as if the right palm is scooping underneath.

3. Then open up again, pointing the right hand toward the ceiling. Repeat a few times.

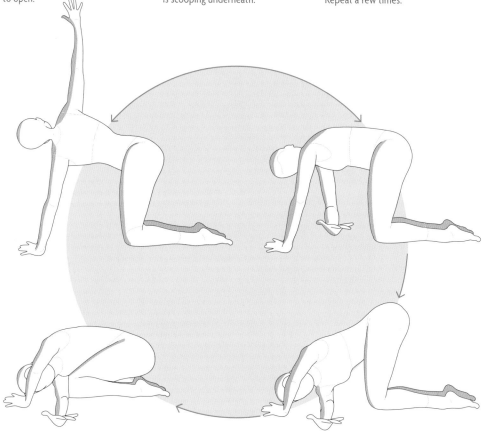

4. On the last repetition, slide the right arm under the left on the floor, bringing the right shoulder and side of the head to the floor.

5. If they don't reach the floor, use a block or blanket under the shoulder/head for support: avoid any pressure through the neck.

6. Relax the right arm and breathe into the back of the twist.

7. To come out, push through the left arm to slide the right arm out. Repeat on the other side.

▶ Superman

1. In All Fours, extend the right arm forward, using the muscles of the armpit and mid-back to support the arm.

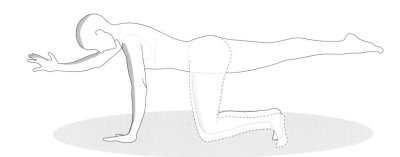

2. If you feel steady, extend the left leg back behind you, using the hips, glutes and hamstrings – not the lower back – to hold up the leg.

3. Flex the back toes of the lifted leg to activate the foot, but don't lock out the knee.

4. Feel the integration from the contact with the floor into the torso.

Make Superman More Adventurous!

1. Donkey Kicks: Bend the lifted leg, with the sole of the foot pointing toward the ceiling, then slowly reach the sole upward: feel the glutes engage and pulse.

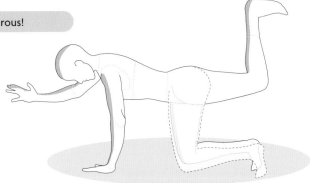

2. Knee to Elbow: Bring the knee of the lifted leg to meet the elbow of the lifted arm under the body: the belly will need to lift and the back will round. Then extend them away again, feeling a gentle lift of the collarbones as you do so. Repeat for several more rounds and then do the other side. You must engage strongly through the contact points with the floor to keep stable.

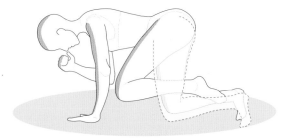

3. Hip Mobility: Bend the lifted leg and open the knee out to the side. Slowly bring the lifted knee toward the supporting elbow, then take it back and extend the leg. Feel the side of the hip engage.

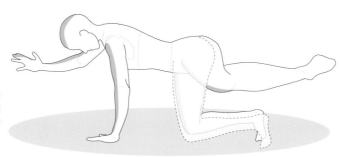

▶ Cow/Cat (*Bitilasana/Marjaiasana*)

1. In All Fours, connect to the sensation dragging your hands toward and slightly away from you, in order to lift the chest and tailbone and look forward. This is Cow.

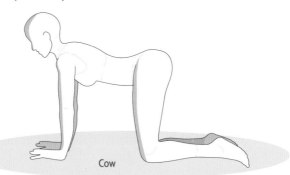

Cow

2. Then push the hands down and pull them slightly inward, with the sensation of pushing the floor away. This allows you to round your back and shoulders. Bring your gaze to your belly button and drop your tailbone. This is Cat.

3. Keep the elbows soft, so they move with the transition. Pay attention to the wave-like quality of the spine as it moves between Cow and Cat.

4. You can add a circular movement to Cow/Cat: start Cow toward your left hand, move back to Cat over the left hip, sideways to Cat over the right hip, then forward to Cow over the right hand. Take the collarbones to the left and continue. Repeat in both directions.

Cat

Child's Pose (*Balasana*)

This is a restorative pose that brings attention to the breath. It can be used as a rest pose at any point in a class, or as an alternative to Down Dog (see page 148).

1. In All Fours (see page 138), move your hips back to your heels. You can have your thighs touching or your knees wider apart.

2. Bring your forehead toward the floor.

3. On each inhale, direct your breath into your back: to the kidney area, ribs and shoulder blades.

4. On each exhale, allow your head and tailbone to become heavy. Avoid pushing; just relax on each exhale.

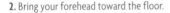
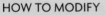

HOW TO MODIFY

- For painful knees, bring the hips forward to release the pressure, or place a rolled-up mat or cushion between the heels and hips.
- If coming forward to the floor is uncomfortable, keep the head lifted, using your hands, a block or a large cushion; or even place the head on a chair.

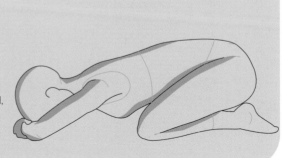

CHANGE IT UP!

▶ Moving Child

1. In Child's Pose, move gently by snaking through the spine, allowing the hips to move from side to side. Wriggle the shoulders, or roll the head against the floor, block or cushion, to release the neck.

2. If the arms are out in front, you can roll them so that the palms face up or down – see how each version feels.

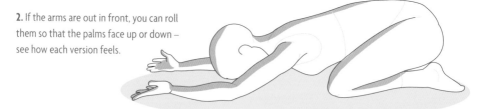

3. Place the arms alongside the lower limbs: be mindful of the neck when you take the support of the arms away.

4. Explore the side body by walking the outstretched arms round to one side and coming up on your fingertips of both hands. Allow the whole body to move with you, including the hip, so that you don't pull on the sacrum.

5. You can gently pulse or rock here to explore the sensation.

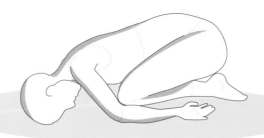

Restorative: Child's Twist

Props: a bolster.

1. Sit with both knees dropped to the right in a zigzag shape.

HOW TO MODIFY

- You can place blocks underneath the elbows and forearms for support, if they are not comfortably reaching the ground.
- If the twist to reach the bolster is too strong, you can raise the height of the bolster by placing blocks underneath it.

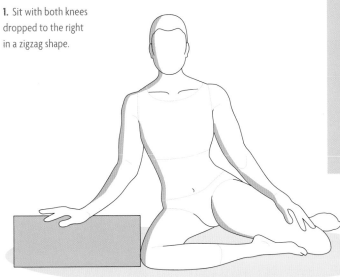

2. Place the bolster on the diagonal beside your right hip.

3. Slowly turn and lower the torso and head to the bolster, hugging it with the arms, with the head turned to the left.

4. Breathe into the back and side of the body.

5. To come up, place the hands to the floor on either side of the bolster and slowly push up.

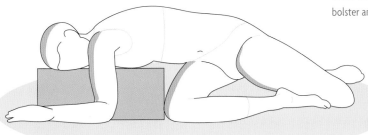

Down Dog (*Adho Mukha Svanasana*)

This a great upper-body strengthener, which
also lengthens the spine.

1. Starting on hands and knees, walk your hands out in
front of you until the arms are active and straight, but
the joints are relaxed. The hands are firmly engaged into
the floor or mat.

2. Move the hips back until the spine feels long.

3. Tuck your toes under and push through the heels to
lift the knees off the ground.

4. Adjust your hands and feet until they feel as though
they are supporting your body weight. This might mean
taking the hands or feet wider apart or changing the
distance between them. Play around until you feel your
body is supported.

5. Practise feeling the connection from the outside
edge of the hand up the arms into the side of the torso.

6. Keep the head and neck soft and gaze at your belly.

7. You can move in Down Dog by pedalling the feet or
moving the hips from side to side.

8. There should be a sense of lightness and buoyancy in
the pose, with nothing locked out or straining.

9. Keep your knees bent as much as you need, to ensure
the spine stays long.

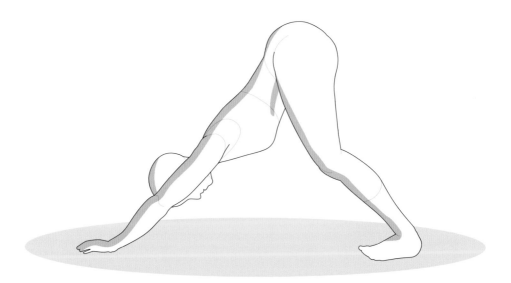

HOW TO MODIFY

- For weak shoulders, wrists and general lack of upper-body strength, do Baby Dog instead. On hands and knees, tuck the toes under and move the hips back toward the heels. Extend your arms away from you, so they are active and the elbows lifted off the floor to lengthen the spine. Engage the hands, side body and tailbone as you would in Down Dog. From Baby Dog, you can come into Advanced Cow/Cat (see page 220).

- Do Down Dog against a table, chair back or wall. Place your hands on a table, chair or wall and walk backward until the arms extend and the spine lengthens. Adjust the position until the hands support the shoulders, and work with your feet until you feel your legs supporting the pelvis. You might come down to 90 degrees at the hips, or higher – especially at the wall. The knees can be soft, or bent as much as you need. Find the outside edges and heel of the hands and explore the connection from here up the arms into the side body. Breathe and lengthen the tailbone.

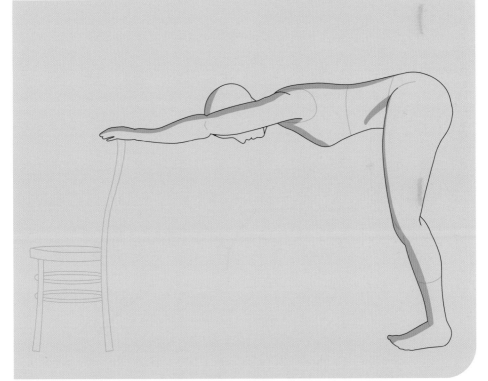

CHANGE IT UP!

▶ Three-Legged Dog

1. From Down Dog, move your right foot toward the left, so that your feet create a three-pointed triangle with your hands. This will enable your pelvis to remain well supported throughout.

2. Lift the left leg up behind you.

3. Strongly connect into the floor with the hands, and allow the shoulders to stay soft.

4. Pulse in and out of the supporting foot.

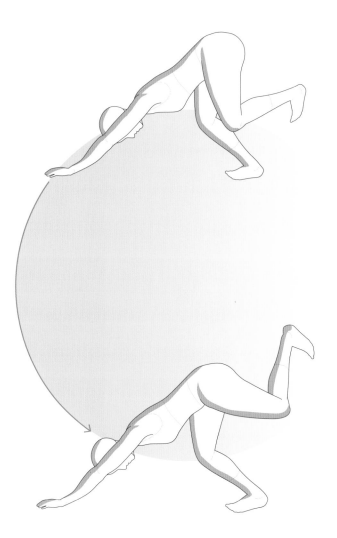

Lamp-Post Dog and Skating Dog

1. From Three-Legged Dog, push into the standing leg and lengthen the lifted leg.

2. Drop the left heel to the right buttock and open the hip. This is Lamp-Post Dog.

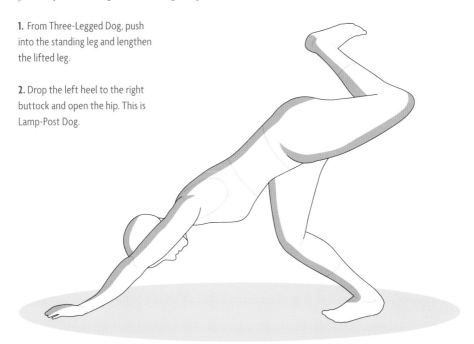

3. Bend both knees and bring the lifted knee behind the standing knee. This is Skating Dog – feel the foot-to-hip relationship.

▶ Elbow Dog

1. From Down Dog, pad through your "front paws" as if you were a dog in its basket.

2. Keep the elbows bent as you lift one hand, then the other, and let your body move with you.

3. As you move from side to side, try lowering one forearm onto, or toward, the floor.

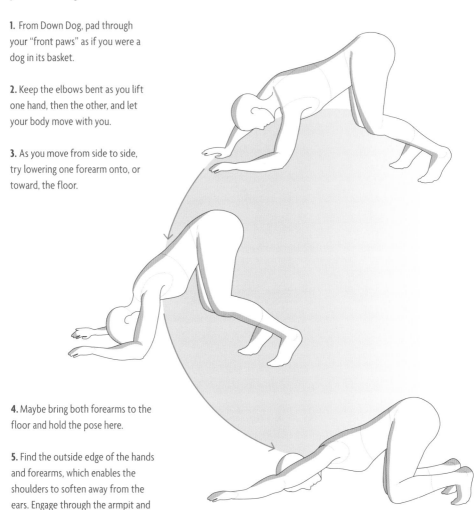

4. Maybe bring both forearms to the floor and hold the pose here.

5. Find the outside edge of the hands and forearms, which enables the shoulders to soften away from the ears. Engage through the armpit and mid-back.

6. Slowly come down into Child's Pose (see page 145) or come back up onto your hands for Down Dog.

▶ Side Dog

1. From Down Dog, come onto the sides of both feet, so that the toes all point in the same direction.

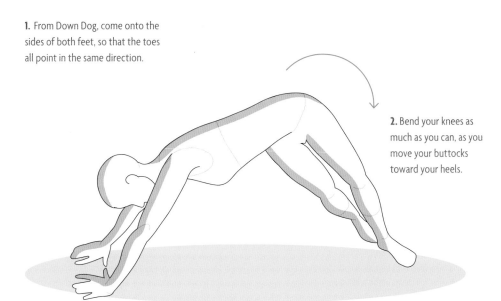

2. Bend your knees as much as you can, as you move your buttocks toward your heels.

3. You can move the hips toward and away from the heels, exploring the lengthening down the side of the back.

4. Keep the neck long and soft.

5. You can come into Rockstar (see page 164) or Popstar (see page 162) from Side Dog.

Floor-Based Front-Body Openers

These poses are ways to open the front body and strengthen the back.

Cobra (*Bhujangasana*)

1. Lie on your front with the hands under the shoulders, palms down, then take them wider than the shoulders, with the elbows lifted.

2. Drag the hands back and away to engage the mid-back; push the tops of the feet gently into the floor, and use these engagements to lift the head, collarbones and maybe the upper chest.

3. Look over each shoulder, roll the chin and release the jaw.

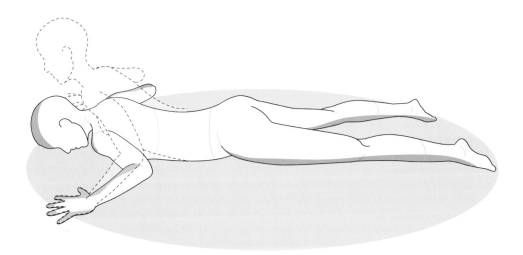

CHANGE IT UP!

▶ Swimming Cobra

1. From Cobra, keeping the chest lifted and the hands dragging back, swim the chest toward one arm and then the other, allowing the head to follow the spine as it moves.

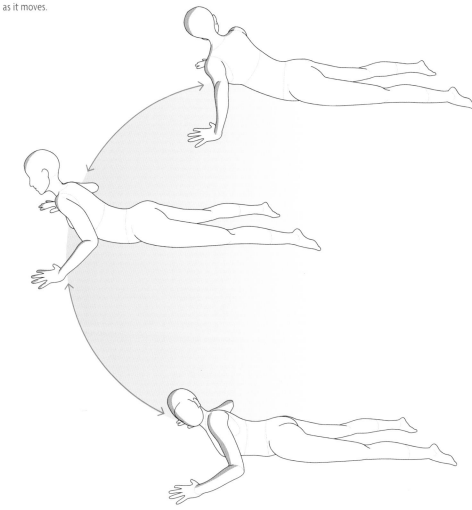

Locust (*Salabhasana*)

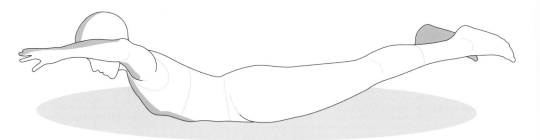

1. In Cobra (see page 154), ensure the mid-back and feet are engaged, then lift the hands off the floor into Locust.

2. You can also lift the legs.

3. Any sensation should be in the mid-back and back of the legs, not the neck and shoulders.

CHANGE IT UP!

▶ Swimming Locust

1. You can progress Locust by swimming: bring the left elbow toward the left ribs and turn to look to that side; then repeat on the right.

2. Ensure engagement is through the mid-back and legs, not lumbar, shoulders or neck.

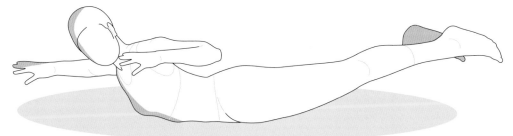

Sphinx (*Salamba Bhujangasana*)

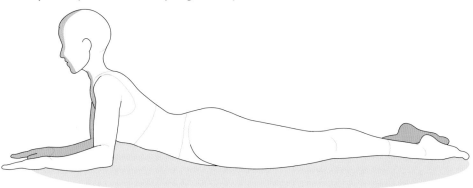

1. In Cobra (see page 154), bring the elbows under the shoulders, with the forearms and hands flat; the fingers can point forward or in whichever direction feels right for you.This allows the chest to lift, and space in the front body.

2. You can roll the chin or turn the head here; maybe wriggle the shoulders or hips.

HOW TO MODIFY

If this feels too strong in the lower back, walk the elbows further forward, but in line with the shoulders, until the ribs come to the floor.

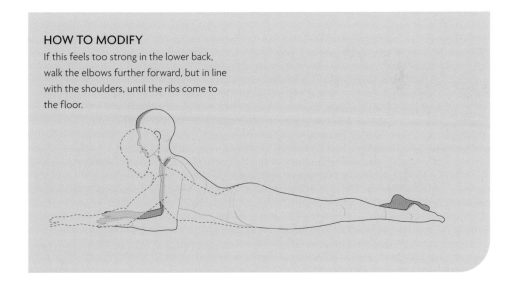

Updog (*Urdhva Mukha Svanasana*)

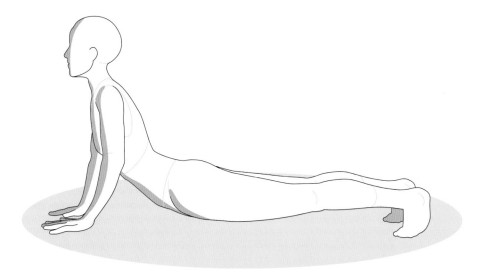

1. In All Fours (see page 138), take the hands slightly further in front and come into Cat position (see page 144).

2. Drag the hands back a little to lift the chest and collarbones and let the hips move forward.

3. Keep a slight bend in the elbows and drag the hands back: the shoulders will drop away from the shoulders and the mid-back will engage.

4. Look forward and avoid throwing the head right back.

5. Push through the heels to stay pliable.

6. The knees can be up or down.

7. Take some swivels from side to side, or circle the hips.

8. To come out, push through the hands and toes to come to Child's Pose (see page 145) or Down Dog (see page 148).

CHANGE IT UP!

▶ Wide-Legged Updog

This is a forceful variation, but is great for strengthening the back.

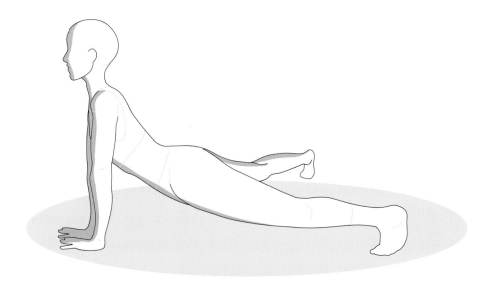

1. Start in Wide-Legged Forward Fold (see page 99).

2. Bend the knees and ensure you have mobility; walk the hands forward until you are in a wide-legged Down Dog (see page 148).

3. Bend the knees, push into the toes and come into a wide-legged Cat position (see page 144) with the knees off the floor.

4. Drag the hands back, lift the collarbones and chest and allow the hips to come forward.

5. Push into opposite heels to create movement through the hips and torso.

6. To come out, bring the knees to the floor, feet toward each other, and move back into a wide-kneed Child's Pose (see page 145).

Front-Body Openers

These poses are all more energetic ways to
open the front body and strengthen the back.

Camel

Camel is a strong pose, so preparation
is needed.

Preparation

1. Kneeling, place the hands on the lower
back and lift the collarbones, take one or
two breaths into the chest, then release.
Repeat a couple of times.

2. Reach the arms forward, then lean
back, hinging at the knees and keeping a
long line from knee to shoulder, until the
legs, trunk and back engage to support
you: you'll feel when it's far enough. Take
a couple of breaths, then reach forward
to come back upright.

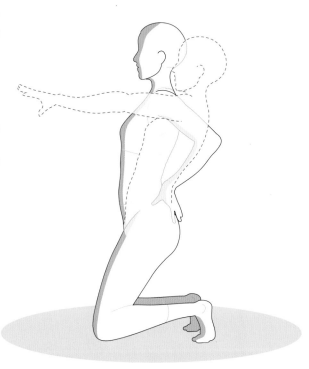

Full Camel (*Ustrasana*)

1. From Camel Preparation, place the hands on
the lower back, lean back from the knees and lift
the collarbones.

2. Feel a sense of lifting up through the ribcage, and
the front of the thighs opening.

3. You may reach behind the thighs to place one or both
hands on the heels.

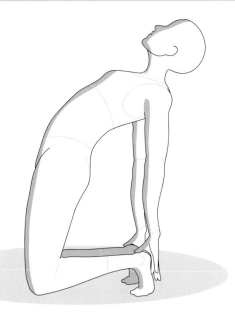

HOW TO MODIFY

- A block can be placed under
  the feet, with the toes
  tucked, to raise the heels to
  meet your hands.
- Alternatively, place two
  bricks or sturdy blocks
  behind you and reach back
  for these.

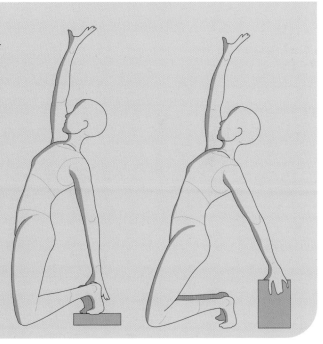

Popstar

1. Sitting, step the left foot forward until it is flat, with the knee over the ankle; the right foot is tucked in.

2. Bring the right hand behind you, so that it supports the right shoulder, but does not jam the shoulder joint.

3. Push into the supporting hand and left foot to lift the hips upward.

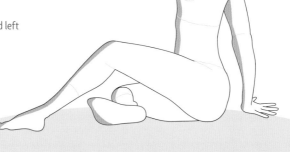

HOW TO MODIFY
If pressure on the supporting knee is too much, try this version:
- Take a Low Lunge (see page 104), with the right leg forward, the chest lifted and the back ankle swung inward.

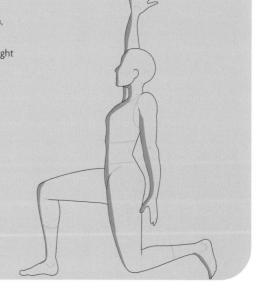

4. Shift the weight between the right hand and left foot; lower and lift the hips; keep the supporting elbow slightly bent.

5. Open the chest and reach back with the lifted arm: breathe into the chest and feel the back engage to support this.

6. Sit down to rest, when needed.

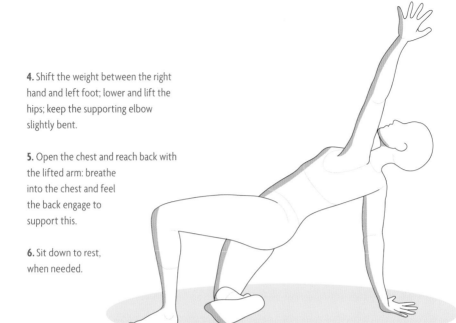

- Place the left hand on the lower back for support, and ensure the front foot is engaged by pushing down; lift the right arm, opening the chest, and reach back a little.
- Push into the front foot to stay stable, and reach up and back.

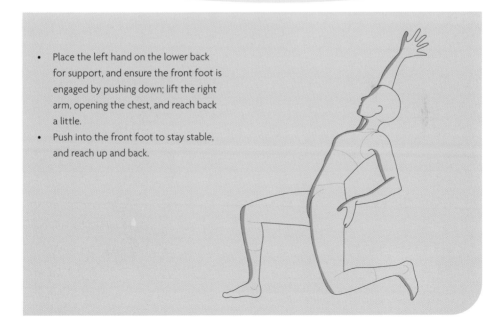

Rockstar

As the name implies, this is a more hardcore
version of Popstar (see page 162).

1. In Down Dog (see page 148),
facing the back of the mat,
get really pliable, with the
knees bending.

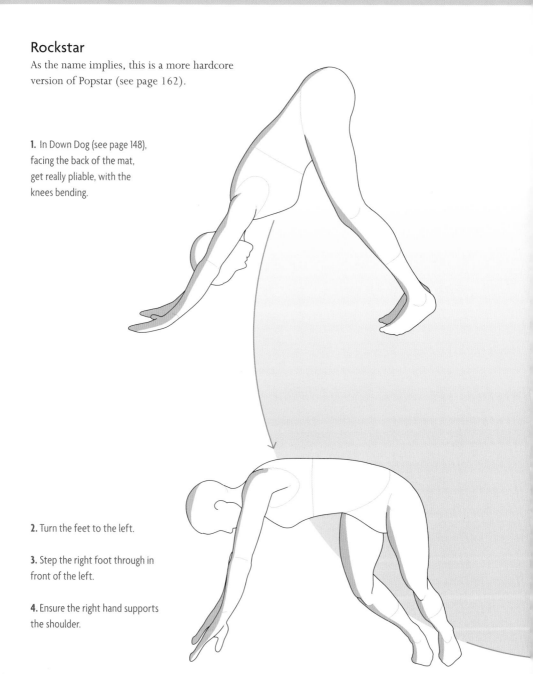

2. Turn the feet to the left.

3. Step the right foot through in
front of the left.

4. Ensure the right hand supports
the shoulder.

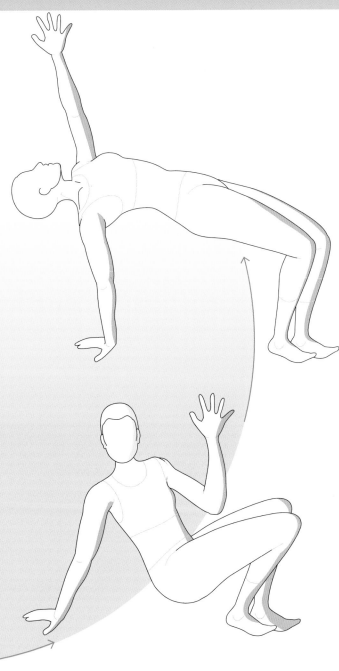

5. Keeping the hips low, start to turn the feet toward the right, unwinding the legs until the feet point to the back of the mat, knees to the ceiling and the whole front of the body points upward. (At this point you can even sit down if you like!)

6. Make sure the supporting hand and feet are in a place where you can push through them to lift the hips up toward the ceiling, open the chest and reach back with the lifted arm.

7. Shift the weight from foot to foot and from hand to feet, lowering and raising the hips. The more you shift, the less weight will drop into the supporting wrist, and the more the whole back line of the body will engage.

Bridge Options

Bridge is a floor-based front-body opener. It is a great antidote to our sitting lifestyles.

Basic Bridge (*Setu Bandha Sarvangasana*)

1. Lie on your back, bend your knees and plant your feet.

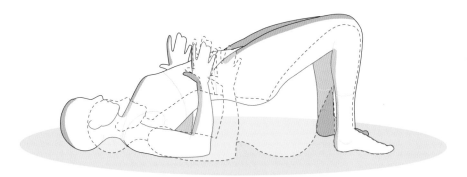

2. Find a place for your feet that isn't too close to your buttocks, but doesn't feel as if the feet are sliding away from you.

3. Push down and imagine the feet are superglued to the mat, so they don't move; however, you can shift weight into the toes, then try to suck the heels back in toward you.

4. When you draw the heels back, you will feel the back of the legs and your buttocks engage.

5. The weight in the heels will cause a slight arch in the lower spine away from the floor.

6. Make "robot" arms, bringing the elbows into the sides of the torso and pointing the fingertips at the ceiling.

7. Push down through the back of the elbows to lift the chest slightly; your hips should stay on the mat.

8. You can now feel a whole "bend" through your back, without even lifting up off the floor! To get more of a bend, you need to lift your hips.

9. Push down through the feet and lift the hips toward the ceiling.

10. Keep shifting the weight through the feet to find a good supportive position: one where the front of the body can open, the feet are fully grounded and the thigh bones are not jamming into the hips.

CHANGE IT UP!

▶ Wide-Legged Bridge

This is the same as Basic Bridge, except that you start by deliberately placing the feet wide. Notice the different sensations around the hips, glutes and pelvis.

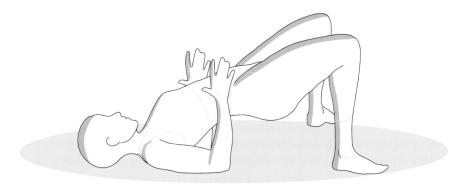

1. Lie on your back, bend your knees and plant your feet wide, turned out and with the knees bent in the direction of the toes.

2. Find a place for your feet that isn't too close to your buttocks, but doesn't feel as if the feet are sliding away from you.

3. Push down and imagine the feet are superglued to the mat, so they don't move; however, you can shift weight into the toes, then try to suck the heels back in toward you.

4. When you draw the heels back, you will feel the back of the legs and your buttocks engage.

5. The weight in the heels will cause a slight arch in the lower spine away from the floor.

6. Make "robot" arms, bringing the elbows into the sides of the torso and pointing the fingertips at the ceiling.

7. Push down through the back of the elbows to lift the chest slightly; your hips should stay on the mat.

8. You can now feel a whole "bend" through your back, without even lifting up off the floor! To get more of a bend, you need to lift your hips.

9. Push down through the feet and lift the hips toward the ceiling.

10. Keep shifting the weight through the feet to find a good supportive position.

▶ Bound Angle Bridge (*Baddha Konasana*)

This activates through the outside edges of the feet. If you have hip, sacrum, knee or lower-back issues, approach with caution.

1. Lie on your back and bring the soles of the feet together, with the outside edges on the mat and the knees dropping wide.

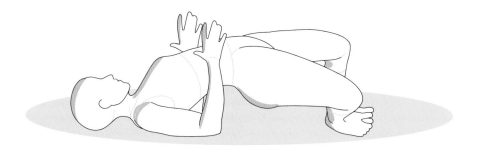

2. Make "robot" arms, bringing the elbows into the sides of the torso and pointing the fingertips at the ceiling.

3. Push down through the back of the elbows to lift the chest slightly; your hips should stay on the mat.

4. You can now feel a whole "bend" through your back, without even lifting up off the floor! To get more of a bend, you need to lift your hips.

5. Push down through the outside edges of the feet and lift the hips up.

6. You need to keep actively engaging the outside edges of the feet. You will feel an openness in the hips, but the buttocks working hard!

Restorative: Supported Bridge

Props: blocks or a bolster.

1. Lie on your back. Place a blanket underneath the head and shoulders for support, if necessary.

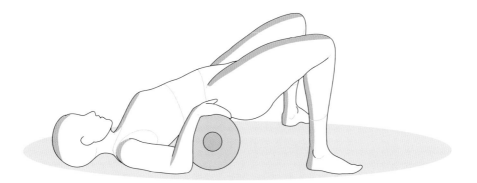

2. Lift the hips into a Bridge position. Slide the blocks or bolster underneath the back of the pelvis.

3. Adjust the feet until you can give all your weight to the floor and the props.

4. The arms can be by your side or overhead, as feels right for you.

5. Practise breathing into the front, side and back of the body.

6. To come out, lift the hips and slide the props out, then lower to the floor.

Seated Poses I

These can be harder to access as the hips are fixed to the ground, which limits our range of movement. Use props to sit on to help free up the body where needed.

Easy Pose (*Sukhasana*)

This seated pose is not always easy! See the modifications to make this pose work better for you.

1. Cross one shin in front of the other, with the heels moving under the opposite knee. You may find it feels more comfortable with one or the other shin in front.

2. Rest your hands on your thighs or knees, but resist pushing or pulling against the legs.

3. Sitting up tall with a long spine, find equal space in the front and back of the body. Relax your neck and shoulders.

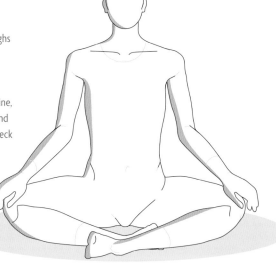

HOW TO MODIFY

If you feel any discomfort in the hips or knees, if the knees are much higher than the hips or if the feet are going to sleep, try the following modifications:

- Sit on a block or cushion. You could also sit on a chair, especially if meditating.

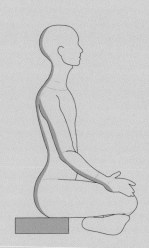

- Straighten out one leg slightly wider than the hip, leaving the other folded in. Have the knee of the straight leg slightly bent.

- Straighten out both legs in front, slightly wider than the hips, with the knees bent a little.

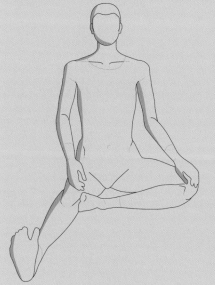

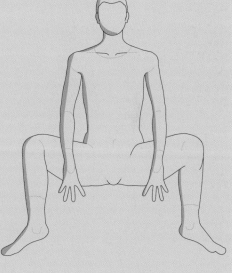

CHANGE IT UP!

Sitting becomes much more interesting when we move. Pages 179–183 have various arm movements that work well in sitting; alternatively, you can add one or two of the following.

▶ Seated Cow/Cat

1. Bring the hands to the knees or thighs and start to round through the spine, tilting the tailbone down and tucking in the chin. This is Cat.

2. Reverse this by tilting the pelvis forward and lifting the chest. This is Cow.

3. Move between the two positions, following the breath, noticing the range of movement and the relationship through the spine and pelvis.

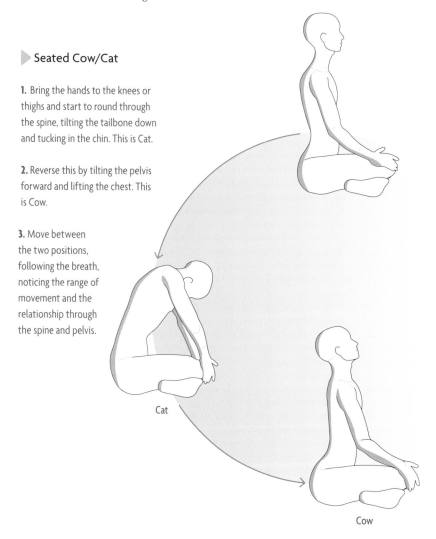

Cat

Cow

Seated Side Bend

1. From a neutral spine, bring the left hand to the floor away from the side of the thigh. When you lean to the left, the hand is in a place where it supports your weight, without the left shoulder creeping up toward the ear.

2. Take the right arm over the top ear and lengthen through the right-hand side of the body. The right buttock can come with you as you reach. Breathe into the side body.

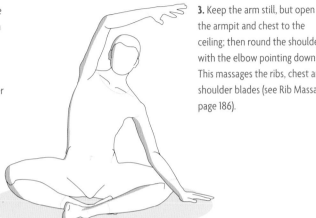

3. Keep the arm still, but open the armpit and chest to the ceiling; then round the shoulder, with the elbow pointing down. This massages the ribs, chest and shoulder blades (see Rib Massaging, page 186).

Seated Twist

1. Find a neutral spine and slowly twist to the right, bringing the right hand behind you.

2. You can move your left hip and put more weight into the right buttock if you feel any pulling on the back of the pelvis or into the lower back.

3. Place the left hand on the right knee or inside the left thigh, but avoid pulling or pushing yourself further into the twist.

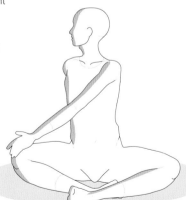

4. You can negotiate the pose by very slowly snaking the spine.

5. Finish by looking over each shoulder, rolling the chin and finding a comfortable place to rest.

6. Breathe into the exposed part of the body.

▶ Shoelace (*Gomukasana*)

This provides a variety of options to take a seated pose into a deep hip extension or to sit more comfortably for movement.

1. Full Shoelace: In Easy Pose with the right leg in front, bring it further round toward the left hip. Then bring the left foot round to the right hip, so the knees are stacked on top of each other.

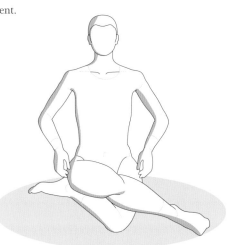

2. Half Shoelace: The Full Shoelace can be tough on the bottom knee: if there is any pain, extend the bottom leg out in front of you.

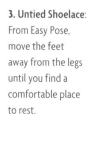

3. Untied Shoelace: From Easy Pose, move the feet away from the legs until you find a comfortable place to rest.

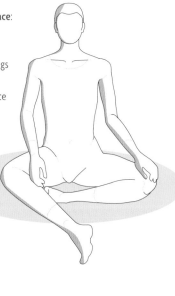

Seated Forward Fold (*Paschimottanasana*)

1. In Easy Pose (see page 170), bring the legs out in front, slightly wider than the hips, with the knees bent.

2. Drape yourself over, or in between, your thighs. The head can hang or you can hold it, resting the elbows on the thighs. Release the jaw, roll the chin and then relax.

3. Breathe into the back body.

4. If comfortable, the legs can be lengthened. Pay attention to any pulling in the lower back.

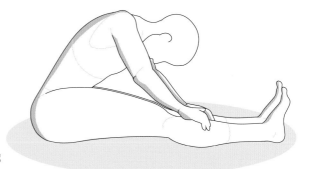

HOW TO MODIFY
You can make Seated Forward Fold a restorative pose by resting the head on a bolster.

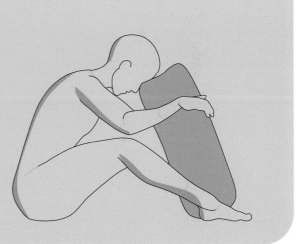

Seated Poses II

These all start in Easy Pose (see page 170); sit on a block, if needed. Use the twists and shapes to create space to breathe into the torso.

Seated Head-to-Knee Pose (*Janu Sirsasana*)

1. Extend the right leg to the side, so that the leg is long.

2. Bend the right knee a little or a lot, or move the left foot further away from your groin, if needed. You can place a block or cushion under the bent knee, especially if it is hanging in the air.

3. If the right leg is straight, keep a micro-bend in the knee to avoid extending through the joint.

4. Activate the right foot by pushing gently down into the floor with the heel.

5. You can add some of the arm movements or a twist from pages 179–187, or fold over the extended leg.

6. Pay attention to the relationship of the pelvis to the spine as you move.

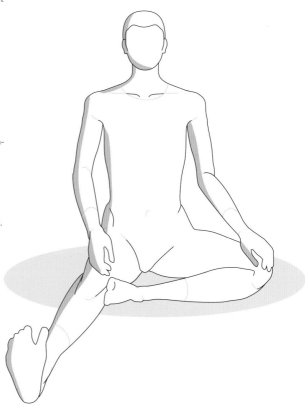

Half Lord-of-the-Fishes Pose (*Ardha Matsyendrasana*)

1. Sit with the legs outstretched in front of you.

2. Step the left foot to the outside of the right thigh, so that the left knee points upward.

3. Gently hold onto the lifted left knee with the right hand, but avoid pulling yourself into the twist.

4. Slowly twist your torso toward your top knee, placing the left hand behind you.

5. Explore the sensations of the twist by turning the head, moving the shoulders and spine a little.

6. To take the pose further, bend the right knee and slide your right foot to the outside of your left hip. If this is uncomfortable, keep the right leg straight.

7. You can also twist away from the upright bent knee by placing the right hand behind you.

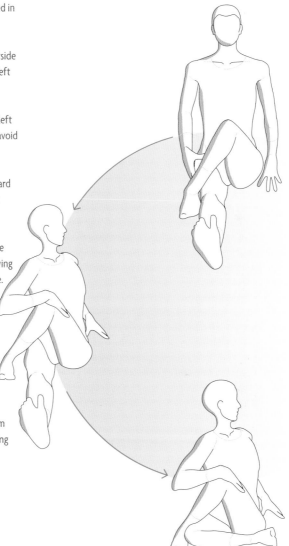

Marichi's Pose (*Marichyasana*)

This twist explores range of movement through the back, sides and front of the torso. Do both versions and notice the difference in engagement and relaxation in the body.

Active Marichi's Pose

1. Bend the left knee and bring the foot in toward the right buttocks and firmly ground it. Push with the outstretched heel, so the pelvis is engaged.

2. Lift the arms into Cactus Arms (see opposite) and slowly twist toward the bent knee and then away from it, turning to the other side. Repeat two to three times in each direction.

3. Feel the muscles in the legs and trunk working to support you.

Passive Marichi's Pose

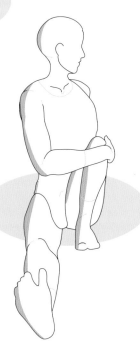

1. Bend the left knee and bring the foot in toward the right buttocks and firmly ground it. Push with the outstretched heel, so the pelvis is engaged.

2. Twist to the left, place the left hand behind you and the right hand onto the bent knee.

3. Explore the sensations of the twist by turning the head, moving the shoulders and spine a little.

Exploring Different Arm Movements

The following arm positions and movements can be added to many seated, kneeling and standing poses to allow further exploration. Examples of how to introduce them with other poses are included below.

In all the arm positions you can explore further by adding gentle movement: keep the arms still and turn the head in either direction; make circles with the torso, allowing the neck, spine and hips to move; and pause somewhere that feels interesting or useful, and take a few breaths before moving on.

Cactus Arms

These can be used in Lunges (see pages 104–110), standing, sitting, Horse Pose (see page 123) and Bound Angle Pose (see page 204).

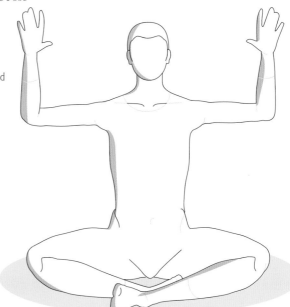

1. Take the arms out to the side and bend the elbows 90 degrees.

2. Keep the elbows at shoulder height and pretend you are dragging the hands back against a wall in front of you.

3. Feel the engagement across the mid-back and under the armpits.

4. If the neck and shoulder-heads get tense, relax, shake it out and try again.

Eagle Arms (*Garudasana*)

Great for opening the shoulders, upper and mid-back, Eagle Arms can be added to the seated Easy Pose (see page 170) or Horse Pose (page 123), or included in Lunges (see pages 104–110) and Warriors 2 and 3 (see pages 100 and 114).

1. Take the arms out wide, then bring them together, placing the right elbow on top of the left, with the fingertips pointing to the ceiling and the backs of the hands touching.

2. You may be able to link finger and thumb or palms together; if not, grab a strap or belt, so there is tension between the hands.

3. Keep the elbows lifted as you explore some of the gentle movements described on page 179.

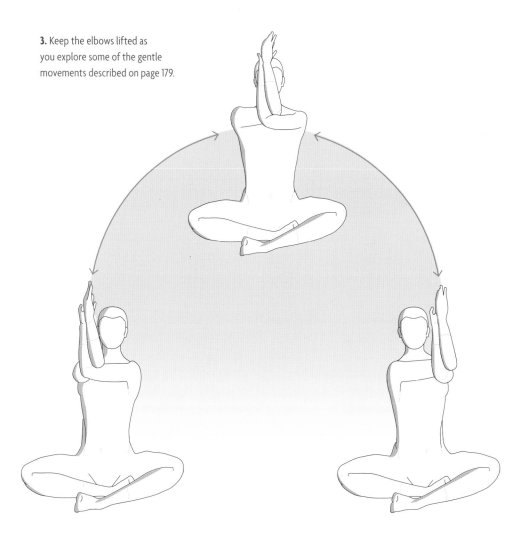

Cow-Faced Shoulder Opener (*Gomukasana*)

This pose is great for desk workers and breast-feeding mothers: anyone whose chest is closed for long periods. You can do this pose kneeling, sitting, standing or even on a chair. It could also be added to a lunge.

Preparation

1. Take the right arm out to the side and explore some arm circles, getting the shoulder-head and shoulder blade to move. Notice the rotation of the arm: how the palm can face in different directions.

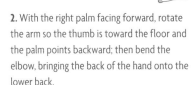

2. With the right palm facing forward, rotate the arm so the thumb is toward the floor and the palm points backward; then bend the elbow, bringing the back of the hand onto the lower back.

3. Now warm up the left arm with some similar arm circles and rotations.

4. In both cases, turn the head slowly from side to side before you explore any movement through the spine.

Baby Cow

1. Use the left hand to gently encourage the right hand across the lower back, until the right forearm rests there and the right hand pokes out to the side of the left waist.

2. Interlace the fingers, make a fist and draw the elbows together.

3. Breathe into the chest and shoulders.

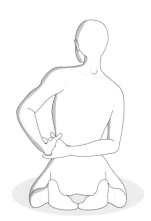

Full Cow

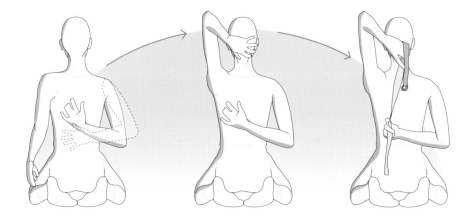

1. Snuggle the fingers of the right hand so they point up between the shoulder blades.

2. Drop the left hand behind the neck, with the left elbow pointing to the ceiling.

3. Interlace the fingers, or grab your shirt with both hands, or use a strap between them – or simply cradle the back of the head with the left hand.

4. Breathe into the chest and shoulders.

Spirals and Side Bends

These work really well seated in Easy Pose (see page 170) or in a Low Lunge (see page 104), with the back leg pointing inward slightly for balance and the hips open to the side a little. They also work standing and in a High Lunge (see page 107).

1. Sitting in Easy Pose with the left shin in front of the right one, place the left hand down on the floor slightly away from the left hip.

2. Reach the right arm over the top of the right ear, leaning to the left, opening up the right-hand side of the torso. Pay attention that the left elbow remains slightly bent, so there is space between the left shoulder and ear.

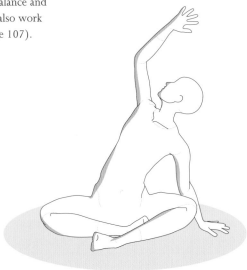

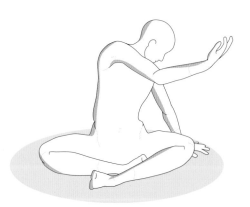

3. Sit up and reach the right elbow across the body toward the left knee, as if offering a plate of food, allowing the spine to round slightly and the chin to drop; the hand doesn't need to touch the knee or even get anywhere near it – it's just the direction of travel.

4. Sit up and alternate between the two arm movements in steps 3 and 4.

5. Place the left hand or forearm onto the left thigh and start with the side bend, then spiral the right elbow toward the left knee.

6. Alternate the between the two arm movements in step 5. Notice the different knock-on reactions through your side body and back from these two movements.

7. Bring the right shin in front of the left one and place the right hand down on the floor slightly away from the right hip. Repeat steps 2–6 with the left arm raised.

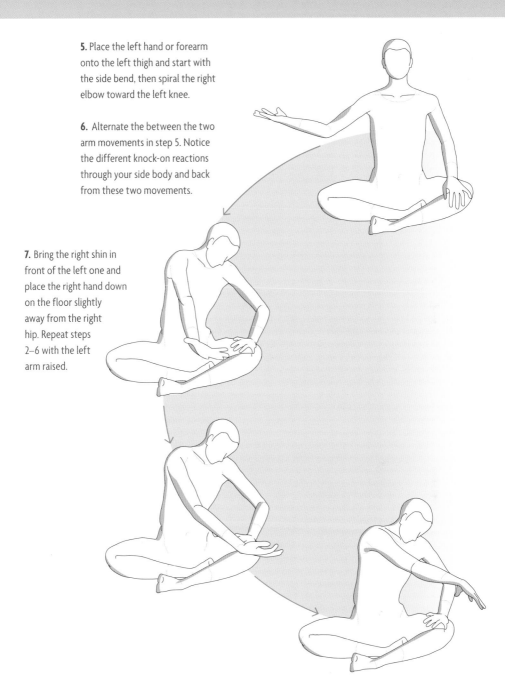

Rib Massaging

This adds an internal massage to all the muscles around the rib cage, increasing our mobility in the mid-thoracic. This can be done sitting or in Side Plank A (see page 134).

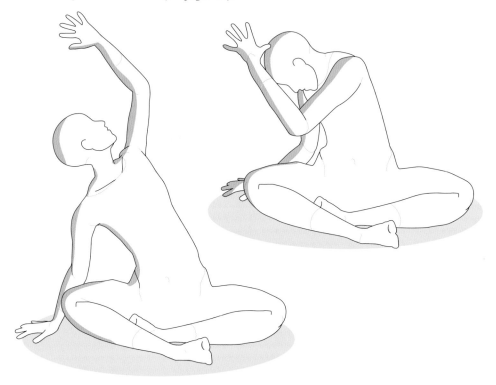

1. In a Seated Side Bend (see page 173), keep the lifted elbow bent and slowly take the elbow back, opening up the armpit and collarbones and maybe looking at the ceiling.

2. Then round the shoulder, directing the elbow at the opposite knee: it won't touch the knee, it's just a direction of travel! Point the chin down.

3. Move between these two positions, noticing the effects around the ribs and shoulder blade.

4. Pause occasionally to breathe into the space you have created through the upper chest or back.

Interlacing Hands Behind and Reaching Back

This can be done kneeling, in Child's Pose (see page 145)
or in a Forward Fold (see page 98).

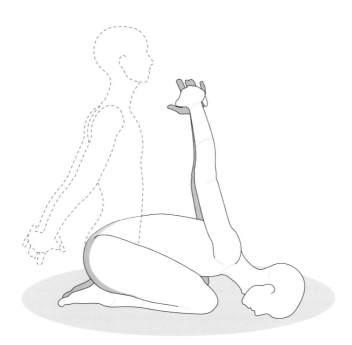

1. Reach the hands behind you, palms up: notice the engagement of the back to lift the hands.

2. You can stay here or interlace the fingers behind you, to further open the chest and shoulders: move the hands from side to side, rolling the head gently.

3. Try with opposite fingers interlaced, and notice any difference through the arms and across the shoulders.

Pigeon Options (*Eka Pada Rajakapotasana*)

Due to the deep external rotation of the front hip, Pigeon
can be delicious for some, painful for others or completely
inaccessible. These versions will hopefully offer alternatives,
so that pigeon becomes feasible for most practitioners.

Active Pigeon

This maintains your active connection to the floor
through the feet and allows you to open the hips,
without dumping weight through them.

1. From Down Dog (see page 148), bring
the left knee forward in line with the left
wrist, then aim the left shin more toward
being parallel with the front line of mat:
this will depend on the bone structure
in your hip.

2. Use the back toes to help the back
leg lengthen behind. Keep the back toes
tucked under to activate the back leg.

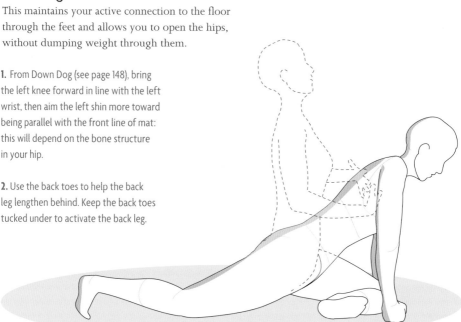

3. Bring the hands toward the
shoulders, so the chest is lifted,
with open collarbones; the hands
can be on blocks, if needed.

4. Using the contact of the toes
with the floor, make circles with
the back heel and notice the effect
up the back leg into the pelvis.

5. You can also circle the hips,
snake the spine, roll the chin:
all these will create knock-on
sensations through the pelvis and
into the left buttock and front of
the right hip. Go in both directions.

6. You can play with lifting one
or both arms: notice where the
engagement comes from.

7. To come out, gently roll your
hips to the left until you end
up sitting.

Lounging Pigeon

This allows you to relax in the pose without pressuring
the knees or hips.

1. In seated Windscreen Wipers (see page
93), drop the knees to the left. Bring the
left knee forward until it is in front of
the left hip, with the shin parallel to the
front of the mat.

2. Depending on your bone structure,
you may have to lean a little or a lot to
the right for this to happen.

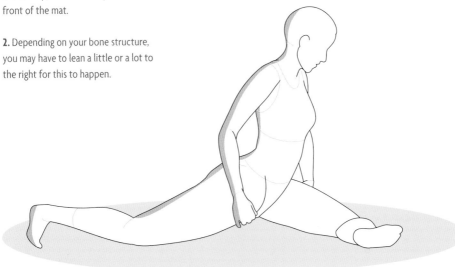

3. Keep the weight on the left
thigh against the floor; use a
blanket under the thigh, if needed.

4. Explore extending the back leg.

5. The back toes might tuck under:
if so, circle the back heel and use
this movement to allow the pelvis
to follow.

6. If the back toes are untucked,
gently circle the pelvis and notice
what you feel through the hips
and legs.

7. Pay attention to the sensations
through the outside of the front
hip and inside of the back hip.

Half Pigeon

1. Like Lounging Pigeon (see page 189), but bring the back knee up to about a 90-degree bend or more.

2. Here you can make hip circles, gently twist from side to side or lift the arms.

3. Just rolling the chin or moving the shoulders can also access sensation in the pelvis.

4. Notice the engagement, if twisting or lifting the arms. Does each side feel the same or different?

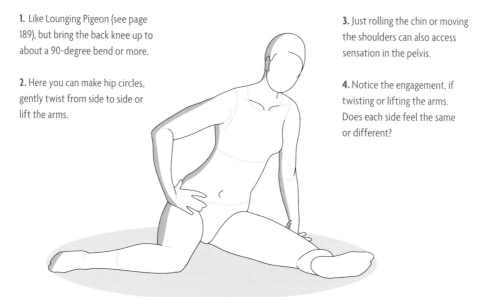

Seated Pigeon

1. Start sitting, with knees bent in front of you. Lean back on your hands and cross the left ankle on top of the right knee.

2. Then bend the right knee until you start to feel sensation through the right buttock and hip.

3. Gently rock from side to side, noticing the effects of the movement on the level and location of the sensation.

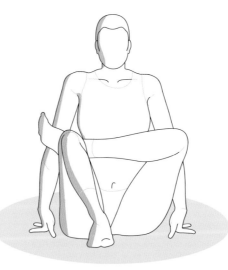

Sleeping Pigeon (*Supta Kapotasana*)

1. Lying on your back, cross the right ankle on the left bent knee and gently rock or pulse from side to side.

2. You can slide the left heel further in toward you, or pick up the left thigh.

3. If the thigh is lifted, make circles with the hips, activating the left hip flexors and releasing the right hip.

4. Reach behind the left thigh and then pulse from side to side. Avoid pulling too much on the back of the thigh: notice the sensation into the side of the hips and thighs.

Wall Pigeon

1. Come into Legs Up the Wall (see page 194).

2. Keep the right leg straight, and cross the left ankle on the right thigh.

3. Bend the right leg a little, so the foot is against the wall.

4. The more you bend the right knee, the closer the leg will come to your chest and the stronger the sensation in the left hip will be.

5. Find your edge and breathe.

Inversions

Inversions can be deeply restorative, so they are a wonderful
way to wind down a practice. These are all gentle inversions,
and you can do a Bridge (see page 166) as well. This book
doesn't include a headstand or handstand because these are
advanced poses that should be taught in person, in a small class.

Half Shoulder Stand (*Sarvangasana*)

This isn't quite a shoulder stand: less pressure rests through the
neck. The upper back is used to support the weight of the legs.

Props: a blanket.

1. Start by having
a blanket folded
twice, under your
head and shoulders
down to the
shoulder blades.

2. Lie down and
bring the knees into
the chest.

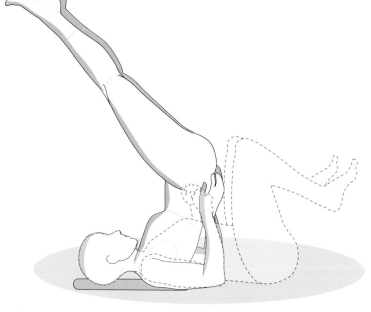

3. Place the hands underneath the
back of the pelvis and keep the
elbows drawn in to lift the hips.

4. Slowly lift the legs toward the
ceiling to roughly a 45-degree angle
over your head.

5. To come out, bring the knees to
the chest and lower the hips.

Supported Shoulder Stand

Props: two blankets and bolster.

1. As for Half Shoulder Stand (see opposite), but place a bolster underneath the pelvis instead of the hands.

2. Lower the hips onto the bolster and raise the legs to the ceiling.

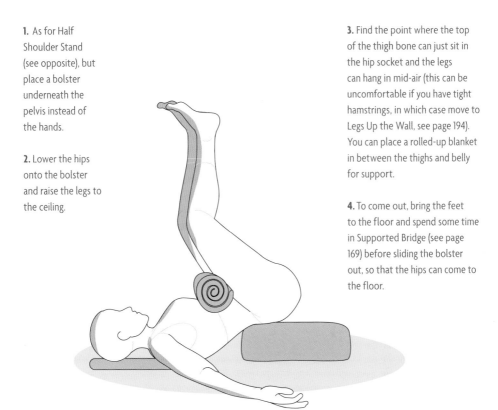

3. Find the point where the top of the thigh bone can just sit in the hip socket and the legs can hang in mid-air (this can be uncomfortable if you have tight hamstrings, in which case move to Legs Up the Wall, see page 194). You can place a rolled-up blanket in between the thighs and belly for support.

4. To come out, bring the feet to the floor and spend some time in Supported Bridge (see page 169) before sliding the bolster out, so that the hips can come to the floor.

Legs Up the Wall (*Viparita Karani*)

Props: a bolster, block or cushion, eye pillow and blanket.

1. Position your mat so that the short edge is against the wall. Have a bolster, block or cushion and eye pillow nearby.

2. Place a folded blanket where your head and upper back will be.

3. Sit down with your right hip flush to the wall.

4. Swing your legs up the wall, as your torso swings out toward the mat.

5. Lay your torso along the mat, with your legs up the wall, and wiggle your buttocks closer to the wall, if needed.

6. Brace your feet against the wall and lift the hips high enough to bring the cushion, bolster or block underneath the hips.

7. You can take the arms overhead or out to the side, or place the hands on the tummy (see *Savasana* options on page 206).

8. Place the eye pillow over the eyes.

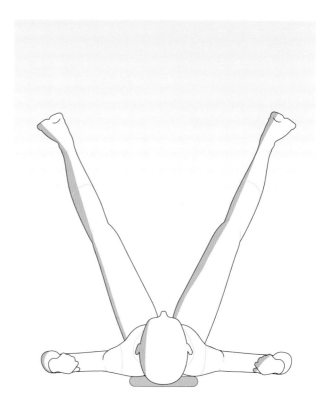

9. To come out, lift the hips to remove the cushion, bolster or block, then bend the knees closer to the chest and carefully roll to the side.

10. Take some time on your side, using the bottom arm as a pillow, before you slowly push yourself to sit up.

HOW TO MODIFY

- Keep the legs straight up against the wall. If the legs don't completely relax, tie a strap around both legs just above the knee, taut enough that the thighs can relax into it.

- Take the legs out wide.

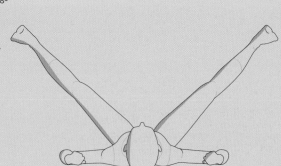

- Bring the soles of the feet together and let the knees drop to the side.

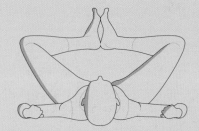

- Using a sofa or chair can be a more accessible option.

CHANGE IT UP!

▷ Wall Twist

You can turn Legs Up the Wall into a twist by:

Props: two blocks.

1. Bending the knees and placing the feet flat against the wall.

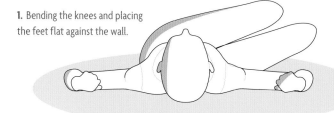

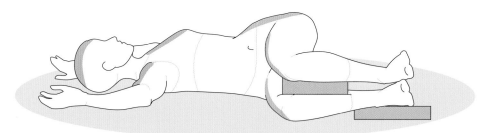

2. Walking the feet round to one side: the knees might come to the floor or need to be propped on a cushion or block. You may need a block between the knees. Keep the shoulders and chest back on the mat.

Supported Fish (*Matsyasana*)

Fish pose is considered the traditional counterpose
to a shoulder stand, as it opens up the front of the
chest, which has just been constricted. You can turn
it into a restorative front-body opener by using props.

Props: a bolster, rolled-up blanket and a cushion.

1. Place the bolster behind you
lengthways, as you sit.

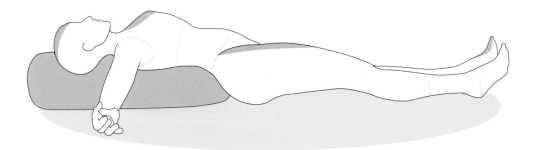

2. Lean back against the bolster:
if that is too strong in the lower
back, you can roll up a blanket
between the back and the bolster.

3. The chin should be pointing
upward a little, but if this is
uncomfortable on the back of the
neck, use a cushion to support the
head in a more neutral position.

4. You can take the arms overhead
or out to the side; the elbows
could be placed on blocks. Be
aware of any pins and needles in
the hands, which means the pose
is too strong and it is time to come
out of the pose.

5. The legs can be straight, bent or
in Bound Angle Pose (see page 204).

6. Breathe into the front of the
chest, armpits and sides of the
neck.

7. If using a block, a smaller blanket
or cushion, this can go under the
shoulder blades, leaning the head
back on the floor. Again use some
support to bring the head into
neutral, if the sensation on the
back of the neck is pinching or
too strong.

On the Back

These poses help to settle the nervous system and can be used to release any residual tension left in the body. Avoid deep stretching and holding for too long at your end-range of motion (see page 45).

Lying Side Bend (*Bananasana*)

1. Lying on your back, take the feet wide and the arms overhead.

2. Take hold of the left wrist with the right hand and gently bend to the right, bringing the left arm overhead. If the shoulders are tight and the arms are hanging in the air, you can use a block or cushion to support them.

3. Cross the left ankle over the right to make a banana shape. Pay attention to any strong sensation in the lower back and lessen the bend if needed.

4. Breathe into the open side of the body.

5. To come out, uncross the legs first, then bring the arms and torso back to central.

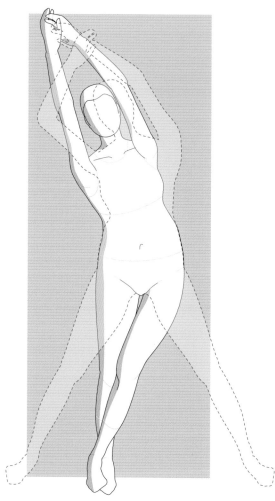

Knees-to-Chest Pose (*Apanasana*)

You can make this pose passive or active, depending on whether you want to release the lower back or start to activate the hips and tummy. This is a good counterpose to Lying Side Bend (see opposite).

Passive Knee-to-Chest Pose

1. Lying on your back, draw the knees to the chest.

2. Clasp the hands around the shins; don't interlace the fingers. Rock gently from side to side and notice how this feels in the back.

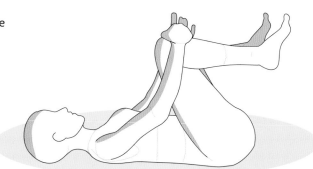

Active Knee-to-Chest Pose

1. Lying on your back, draw the knees to the chest, keeping the arms relaxed.

2. Take the arms overhead or to the side, palms down, and push down to help provide more stability through the torso.

3. Bring the knees into the chest. Use the tummy muscles and side body to rock from side to side; notice how this feels across your back and through the side body.

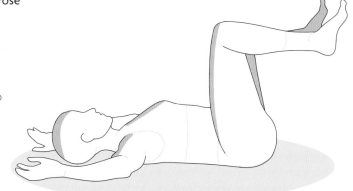

Stronger Abdominal Twist (*Jathara Parivartanasana*)

1. From Knees-to-Chest Pose (see page 199), drop the knees to the floor on the left: you may need a block or cushion underneath them, if the twist is too strong.

2. The knees can move away from the belly button if it is too strong for the lower back.

3. Open out the chest, relaxing the right shoulder to the floor.

4. You can make some arm circles by dragging the back of the hand across the floor from hip to overhead, to find the best place to rest and breathe into the chest and armpit.

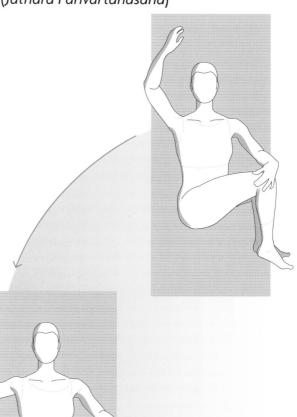

5. The top leg can extend, if that is comfortable: rest it on a sofa edge or block.

6. Notice the relationship from the armpit to the hip and out into the foot.

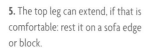

Supine Twist (*Supta Matsyendrasana*)

1. Lying on your back, bring the left knee into the chest and keep the other leg long along the mat.

2. Using your hands, bring the knee across the body and then back out to the side a few times.

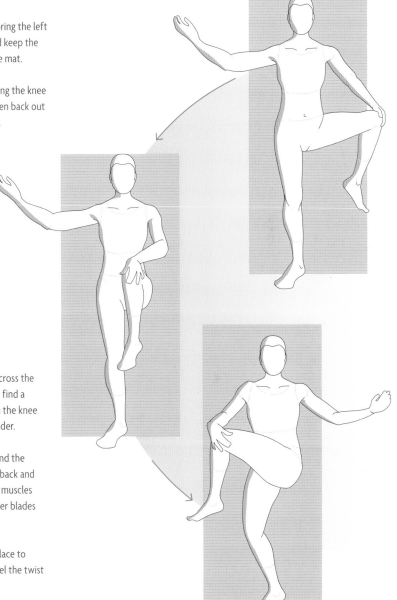

3. Bring the left knee across the body toward the floor: find a balance point between the knee and the opposite shoulder.

4. You are looking to find the twist through the mid-back and side body: think of the muscles underneath the shoulder blades and armpits.

5. Find an interesting place to stop, where you can feel the twist and breathe.

Pigeon Twist

1. Lying on your back, bend the knees and place the left ankle on the right knee in Sleeping Pigeon (see page 191).

2. Rock gently from side to side, or bring the thighs in toward the chest and pulse from side to side (not using the hands will make this more active).

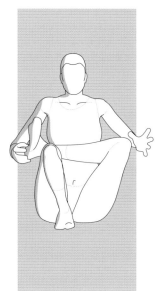

3. Then start to roll to the right until the sole of the left foot hits the floor: you may want a block underneath the foot, to raise the level of the floor.

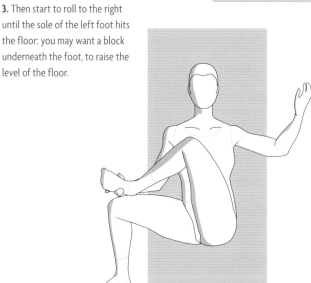

4. Keep the shoulders on the floor and relax: feel into the side of the buttocks.

5. If you feel this in your lower back or across the back of the pelvis, come out of the twist and stay in Sleeping Pigeon.

Happy Baby (*Ananda Balasana*)

This is a traditional hip opener: notice what is happening not only on the back and sides of the hips, but also the compression of the front of the hip flexor. If there is pinching sensation, ease off from the pose. Bound Angle Pose (see page 204) is a good counterpose.

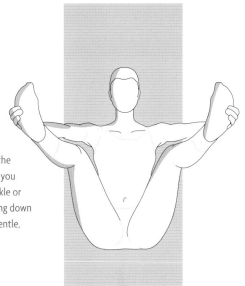

1. Lying with the knees bent, draw them toward the armpits, aiming more for the sides of the torso than the front of the chest.

2. Lift the soles of the feet, so they are facing the ceiling.

3. Hold the back of the knees; you may find you can hold the calf, ankle or foot, but avoid pulling down too much: this is a gentle, releasing pose.

HOW TO MODIFY

- If comfortable, you can rock from side to side. I like to roll to one side and turn it into Lounging Pigeon (see page 189), then roll back!
- Do one side at a time: ground the supporting foot for stability.

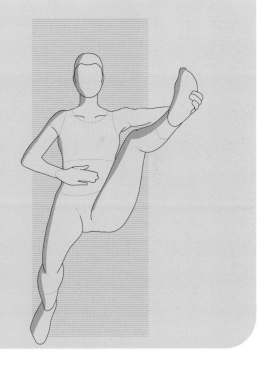

Sleeping Tree and Bound Angle Pose
(*Supta Vrksasana* and *Baddha Konasana*)

This opens the front of the hips. Pay attention to what is
happening across the SI joint in the lower back (see page 80),
as these poses can pull on this area.

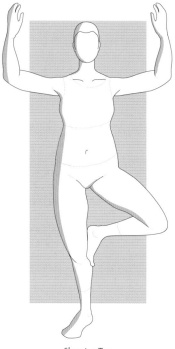

Sleeping Tree

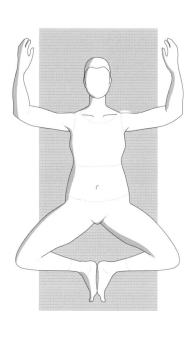

Bound Angle Pose

1. On your back, straighten one
leg out, then bring the sole of the
other foot so that it rests against
the inside of the straight leg: this is
Sleeping Tree – the Tree Pose (see
page 111) on your back.

2. The sole of the foot can be
against the calf, knee or thigh.

3. Bring the soles of both feet
together into Bound Angle Pose,
opening the front of the hips.

4. If you are staying longer than
a few breaths in either of these
versions, you may want to put a
block or cushion under the bent
knee to reduce the impact on the
hip and sacrum.

Tummy Tree and Twist

1. Lying on the belly, bend one knee and bring it up toward the hip.

2. The foot can be toward the leg or away: find whatever position is comfortable.

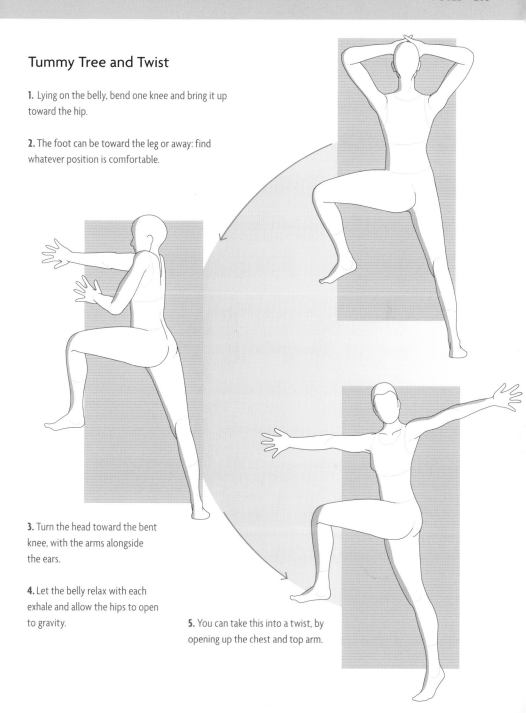

3. Turn the head toward the bent knee, with the arms alongside the ears.

4. Let the belly relax with each exhale and allow the hips to open to gravity.

5. You can take this into a twist, by opening up the chest and top arm.

Savasana Options

Never, ever miss *Savasana*: a resting pose – generally on your back – of total relaxation. Even if you are practising at home, allow five additional minutes for this critical part of your practice. *Savasana* is where your nervous system absorbs everything you have been doing in your session. Not only will the nervous system start to allow healing and regeneration, but this is also where the body and brain imprint the movement and poses. *Savasana* plays a key part in switching on alpha waves in the brain (see page 67), which are where the brain gets important rest from thinking.

Many people find *Savasana* difficult, often due to a busy mind, being uncomfortable lying down or feeling anxious. It can help to do some breathwork or *pranayama* after the physical practices before *Savasana*, to calm the mind. When in *Savasana*, the most simple approach is to give your mind a job to do; here are some ideas.

Complete Body Relaxation

1. Relax the jaw, tongue, eye sockets, eyeballs and the space between the eyebrows. Swallow to relax the throat. Allow the collarbones to move away from each other: you might need to adjust the position of the arms to allow this. Soften the belly. Take your ankles far enough apart so that the feet flop out to the side, enabling the legs and hips to relax.

2. Imagine you are lying on a soft, spongy surface; you are completely supported, but there is some "give" to the floor. Each time you exhale, allow yourself to get heavier and heavier; each time you breathe out, give your body weight to the floor as best you can, imagining it sinking a little into the spongy surface.

3. Softly count the breath, starting again at one if you get distracted. Or you could say, "Breathing in, breathing out."

4. Combine the breath with a visualization or mental image: breathing in, see the breath go down the body to your feet; exhale and visualize the breath going all the way up to your head.

5. Bring one or both hands on your tummy and send the breath into the space underneath: feel the breath moving in the space beneath your hands. As you breathe in, the tummy rises; as you breathe out, the tummy falls.

6. Playing soft music may help, as it provides a gentle distraction. Sometimes complete silence can be difficult, if you are having lots of anxious or negative thoughts.

7. After a few minutes you may find that you can release the "job" you have given your mind to do, and can return to complete rest. Thoughts will come and go, as that is what they do, but can you allow them to pass across the screen of the mind, rather than getting involved in each one.

Traditional Corpse Pose

Props: three blankets, an eye pillow and a cushion.

1. Fold one blanket in half and place it on the mat to protect the sacrum.

2. Lying down, take the ankles quite wide, so that the feet, legs and hips relax.

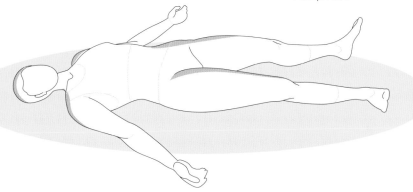

3. A cushion may be needed underneath the head, to allow the chin to come into a neutral position and for the back of the neck to feel long.

4. Drape a folded blanket across your lower belly and pelvis and cover yourself with the third blanket, if needed. Use the eye pillow to cover your eyes.

5. Position the elbows away from the body at about 45 degrees, so you get a sense of the collarbones moving away from each other and the chest opening a little.

HOW TO MODIFY

- To help the lower back, you can bend the knees and take the feet to the edge of the mat. Drop the knees together, so that they are supporting each other. Alternatively, keep the bent knees roughly hip-width apart and secure them with a looped belt. This will enable the knees to relax as you hold the belt. Both options will let the lower back soften to the floor and will also relax the thighs and hips.

- You can also place a bolster or cushions underneath the knees, keeping the ankles wide. This again releases the lower back, but there is no effort whatsoever through the legs now!

Side Lying

Props: a blanket and a cushion or bolster.

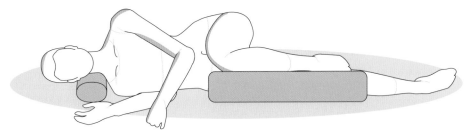

1. Place a blanket on the mat, folded over at least once. Lie down and roll onto your preferred side: you want the blanket underneath the hip bones for comfort.

2. Keep the bottom leg long, bend the top knee and rest it on a cushion or bolster.

3. Use a cushion underneath the head, and have the underneath arm pointing to the long edge of the mat. You can even have some blocks to place the top arm on.

Belly Lying

Props: a blanket.

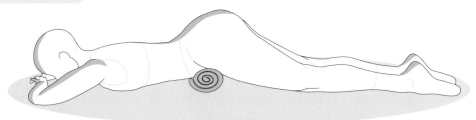

1. Have a folded blanket across the mat to rest your pubic bone on, then bring yourself down to your belly.

2. Find a comfortable place for the legs that works for your hips and lower back.

3. Fold the arms and place the forehead on them, or take the arms forward. Turn the head to one side and place it on the mat: be aware of how your neck feels. Then turn the head to the other side, too.

Reclined *Baddha Konasana* (aka The Armchair)

Props: a bolster, six sturdy blocks, four blankets or soft cushions.

1. Support the bolster on two of the blocks, so it is reclining. The blocks will need to be at an angle.

2. Sit in front of the bolster, with your back up against it.

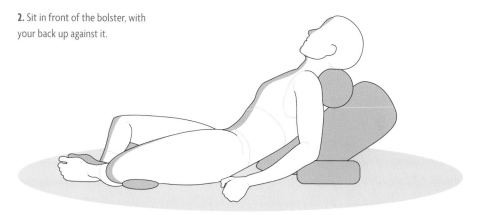

3. Bring the soles of the feet together and allow the knees to drop out to the side: support the knees with rolled-up blankets, cushions or blocks. You do not want the sensation in the hips to be strong, as you will be in the pose for several minutes, so ensure the legs can relax completely and there is not too much pulling on the lower back.

4. The other blocks, with the blankets or cushions on them, should go alongside you, to act like the arms on an armchair.

5. Lie back against the bolster: you may need a cushion or blanket to support the head.

6. Place your elbows and forearms on the "arms" of the chair and relax for 5–7 minutes.

Moving and Transitions

One of the most popular forms of postural yoga is a dynamic form called Vinyasa yoga (see page 14). Some forms of Vinyasa yoga can be quite fast and energetic, whereas there are classes where the flow will be much slower; much depends on the teacher.

Often it is not the poses themselves that cause issues for students, but how we get into them, get out of them and then into the next pose: especially when this is being done quite quickly. The movements are just as important for building strength and flexibility in the body as the poses themselves, and they are also places where people can get injured if not paying attention. In some classes teachers will give students the freedom to move in a way that suits them, so knowing different options will help you decide what will work for you.

In this section we will outline how to do some of the more common transitions that you will find in most yoga classes, and look at what is being engaged and opened in the body as we move. Often the transitional movement can be just as interesting and useful as the actual pose we end up in! Modifications are also provided for these transitions.

In general, remember that movements need stability first! Whatever part of your body is placed on the floor to stabilize you must be engaged and grounded and able to take shifting weight. Secondly, the body cannot move if it is rigid: you need springiness and buoyancy to move, and this comes from bending the knees and elbows. Take your time when moving, there is no rush.

The transitions covered here include moving between standing to a lunge position, moving into a Forward Fold, moving into Down Dog and how to reverse all or part of this process. Also included are options for a linking sequence known as a *vinyasa*, which is a way of flexing and extending the spine to reset the body in between sequences. How to roll up from lying down to seated, and getting from seated to standing are also included.

Some classes will align breath instructions with these transitions: inhaling and exhaling in certain places. This works if your breath and movement patterns match the instructor's, but if they don't it can sometimes feel as if you're holding your breath, or breathing too fast; both of these will kick in the stress response. It is much better to find your own way of breathing, and to ensure you keep breathing through your nose in a soft, steady way. Watch for the breath getting laboured or if it catches or holds: this might be a sign to slow down.

Sun Salutations

The movements included in this book form the basis of sequences known as Sun Salutations. These are included in many, if not most, yoga classes in various different combinations. Sun Salutations are a combination of an old ritual movement of bowing to the sun, with more gymnastic elements added in, such as planks, lunges and even jumping back and forward.

They are used as a warm-up in classical Ashtanga yoga, or are sequenced later in other styles. It is thought that they were developed in the 1920s and 30s from these traditional rituals and the influence of Western gymnastics: when done fast they are sometimes akin to a burpee!

Sun Salutations are not included in this book in their usual form because we are looking at slightly different ways to move – ways that honour our often sedentary 21st-century lives and provide a greater variety of movement and possibilities. You can create your own Sun Salutations from the following movements, starting from standing: stepping back to Lunge (see pages 218–219), stepping back to Down Dog (see pages 214–215), a choice of vinyasa (see pages 220–223) and then reversing it all back to standing. You'll also find that these movements form the basis of the standing sequences in the practices in How to Live Your Yoga (see pages 268–275).

Rolling or Hingeing Down from Standing

Rolling down can be difficult for many people, especially those with lower-back issues, tight hamstrings and limited hip rotation. If you find it difficult, try hingeing instead. To reverse the sequence, bend the knees and push through the feet to engage the whole muscular chain in the legs and buttocks to lift the torso, rather than putting all the pressure in the back to lift up. You can roll or hinge to come up.

Rolling Down

Hingeing Down

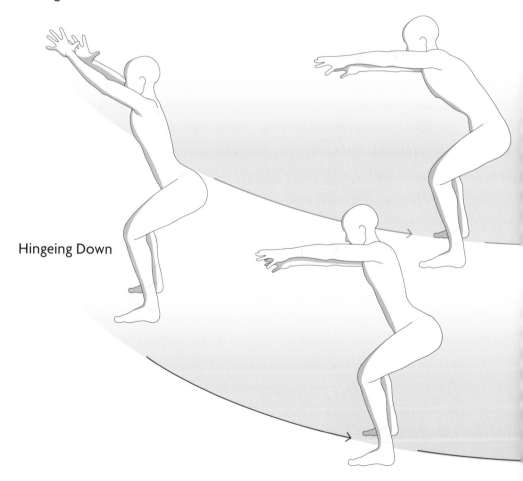

1. Standing in Mountain Pose (see page 97), adjust the feet until you feel the feet and legs are supporting the pelvis and spine. Bend the knees to allow the pelvis to move behind you. Keep the weight in the feet, legs and buttocks, so they bear the weight of the torso coming down, and not the back.

2. As the knees need to bend, the pelvis drops behind the hips and the tummy comes onto or toward the thighs, by rolling the spine or hinging at the hips to keep the spine straight.

3. Bring the hands to the floor, then slowly lift the hips toward the ceiling. You are now in Forward Fold (see page 98).

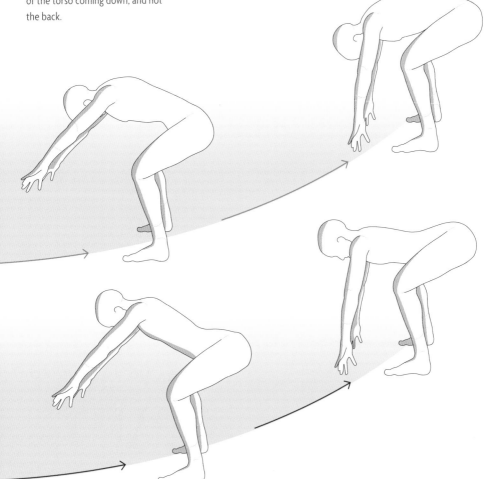

Stepping Back to Down Dog

This involves upper body strength, core engagement and decent hip mobility. You can move through All Fours (see page 138), then into Down Dog (see page 148) as a modification.

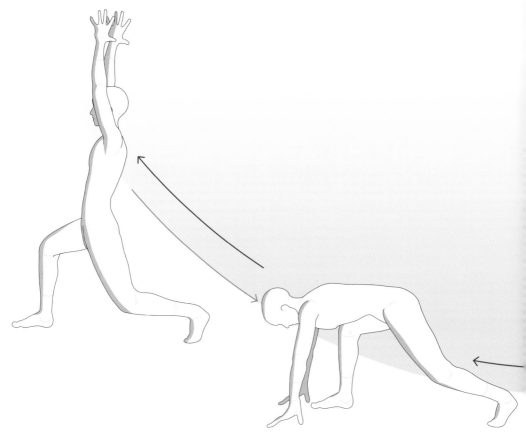

1. Start from any standing pose. This example shows High Lunge (see page 107).

2. Bend both knees deeply. The back knee can come onto the floor.

3. Bring the hands down to the floor about shoulder-width apart.

4. Take the front foot a bit wider, outside the hands.

5. With the back knee lifted, shift the weight between hands and feet.

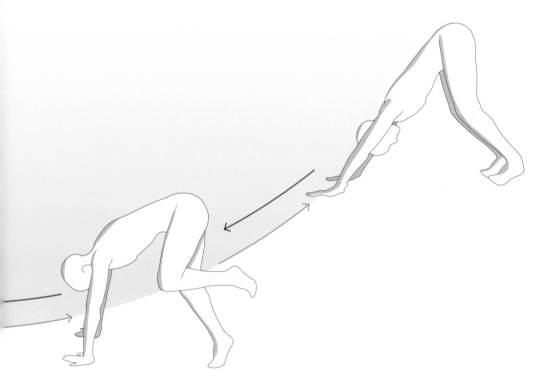

6. Keep buoyant and mobile through the body by pushing the hands into the floor and bending the back knee. Then lift the front foot and step it back to join the other foot behind you.

7. Move the pelvis back for Down Dog (see page 148).

8. If the back knee is on the floor, slide the front knee back to join it, making an All Fours shape (see page 138).

9. Tuck the toes under and come into Down Dog.

Stepping Forward from Down Dog

You may find either walking feet forward or hands toward feet easier for you. Play with both options!

1. In Down Dog (see page 148), keeping the knees bent, start to walk or step the feet towards the hands (or walk the hands back towards the feet) until you are in Forward Fold (see page 98). Walking forward can be done in one step or many.

2. Roll up to a standing pose.

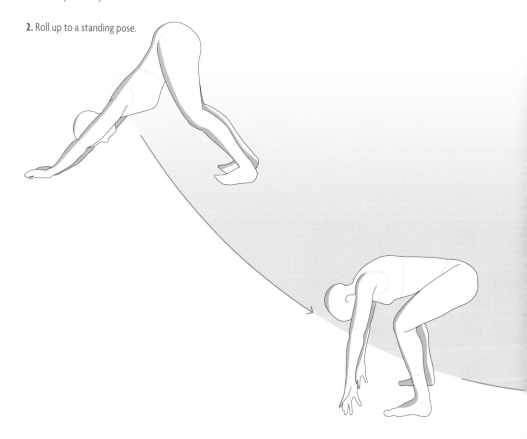

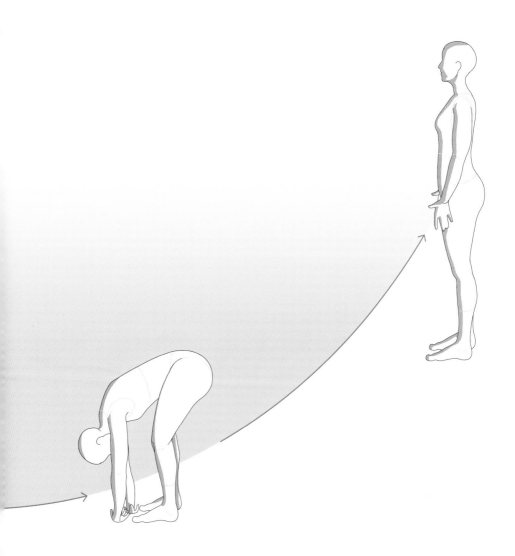

Stepping to and from Lunge

This requires a shifting of weight through the legs and pelvis so remain buoyant and springy in the body.

Stepping back to a lunge (steps 1–5)

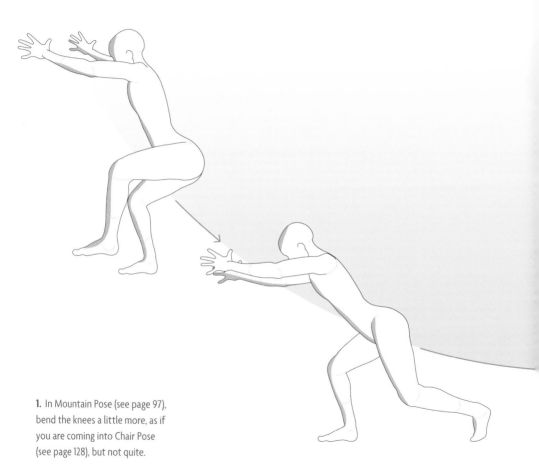

1. In Mountain Pose (see page 97), bend the knees a little more, as if you are coming into Chair Pose (see page 128), but not quite.

2. Shift the weight more into the right foot and lift the left foot off the ground.

3. Keep the standing knee bent as you take the lifted leg toward the back of the mat.

4. Keep the weight in the standing leg until the back toes hit the mat.

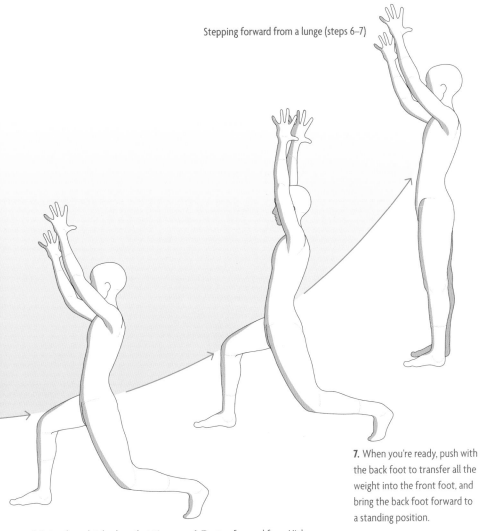

Stepping forward from a lunge (steps 6–7)

7. When you're ready, push with the back foot to transfer all the weight into the front foot, and bring the back foot forward to a standing position.

5. Bring the pelvis back so that it's between the feet, then lift the chest and arms into High Lunge (see page 107).

6. To step forward from High Lunge, keep springy by bending both knees.

Vinyasa Options

A vinyasa is a linking sequence of poses that are used to flex and extend the spine in some way to reset the body, ready for the next part of the sequence. Traditionally this can be quite tough, so here are some options for your vinyasa that give greater mobility and are easier on the wrists and shoulders.

A vinyasa takes you to and from Down Dog (see page 148), so in the examples below, this is your start and finish point.

Cow/Cat

Cow/Cat (see page 144) is the most gentle option, providing a simple way to access an opening of the chest and space across the back.

Advanced Cow/Cat

With Advanced Cow/Cat and the stronger Rolling Vinyasa (see page 222), pay attention to the length between the hands and feet. You don't want the space to be too long or too short. Adjust the feet or hands so that you feel supported.

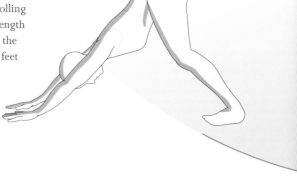

1. From Down Dog (see page 148), lower the knees to All Fours (see page 138), tuck your toes and move your hips back toward your heels.

2. Take the arms further out in front, so that the arms are straight and active.

3. Push through your toes to come up and forward with a rounded back, looking at your belly, in Cat pose.

4. As the shoulders arrive over the wrists, lift the collarbones with a slight dragging back of the hands, and look forward; bring the hips forward as far as feels comfortable into Updog (see page 158).

5. Keep the arms straight, but with a little give in the elbow; the chest is lifted and the shoulders are away from the ears.

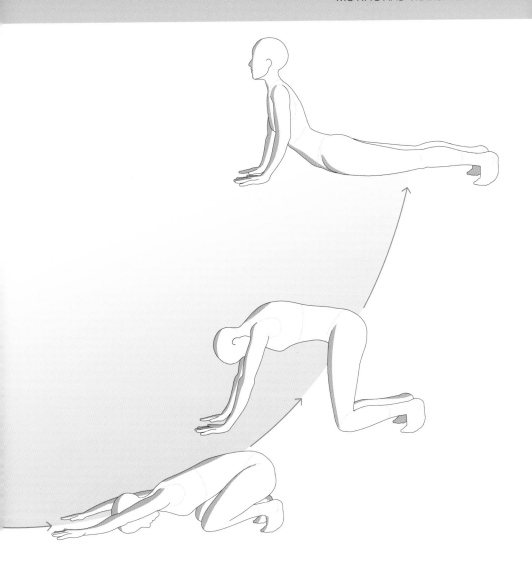

6. You can look over opposite shoulders, snake the spine or move the hips.

7. The knees can come up from the floor, if you wish.

8. Push through hands and feet to come up, with a sense of pushing the hands down and slightly toward each other to round the back and look at your belly.

9. As you move back, soften the knees, push through your heels and come up into Down Dog.

Rolling *Vinyasa*

This is the same as the Advanced Cow/Cat (see page 220), but with more weight-bearing. Remember to use the muscles around the armpit and across the torso, not just the shoulders and wrists.

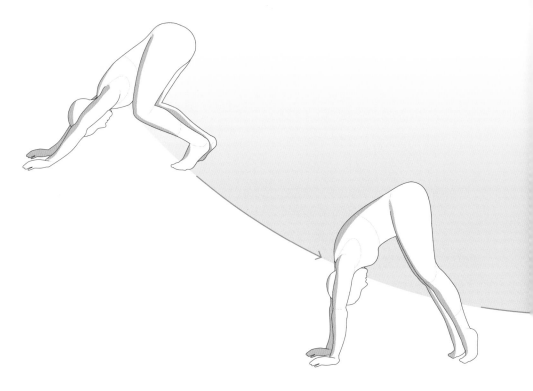

1. In Down Dog (see page 148), bend both knees, bringing your hips toward your heels. Your feet will need to be wide enough for this to happen.

2. Push through the toes, rounding your back and looking at your belly into a long Cat pose (see page 144).

3. As the shoulders arrive right over the wrists, begin a sensation of dragging the hands back as you lift the collarbones, look forward and lower the pelvis toward the floor; the chest stays lifted.

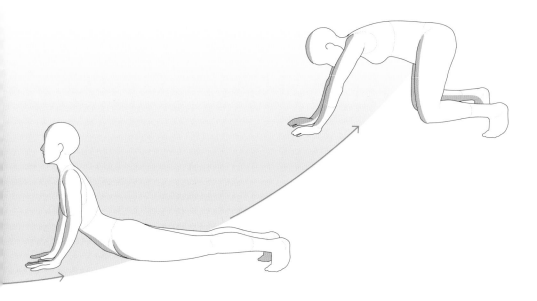

4. You are now in Updog (see page 158): keep strong through the heels, if the toes are tucked under. Alternatively, you can untuck the toes.

5. Tuck the toes under, push through hands and feet to come up, rounding the back and looking at your belly.

6. As you move back, soften the knees as you arrive back in Down Dog.

Rolling Over and Other Movements

Rolling over is one of the first movements we learn as babies, as we play with gravity. In all of these poses the idea is not deep stretching, but simply finding space and then moving on.

Windscreen Wipers

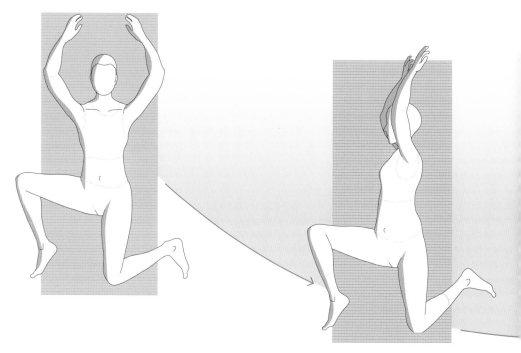

1. Lying on your back, bend the knees and plant the feet on the mat wider than your hips.

2. Take the arms overhead, bending the elbows so that the arms relax on the floor near your ears.

3. Keep your feet wide for this exercise, so there is room for your knees to move.

4. Start by dropping the knees from side to side; they don't have to come all the way to the floor.

5. Pay attention to any sensation through the hips and lower back.

6. When the knees go to the right, reach the left arm away alongside the ear.

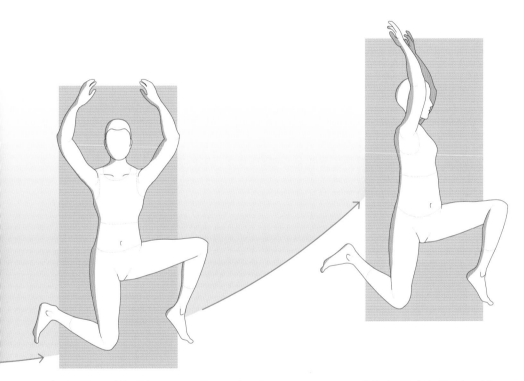

7. The shoulder may lift off the floor slightly, if it feels okay in your back.

8. Repeat on the other side; use the feet to push yourself from side to side a few times.

9. Notice how this movement creates a chain of sensation from the fingertips to the armpit to the ribs, waist and hips, and even into the front of the thigh.

10. Pause with the knees to the right. Bring your left heel closer to your left buttock, with the inside edge of the left foot against the mat.

11. Push with the inside edge of the left foot, engaging the left glutes and lifting the left hip. You can also reach the left fingertips away, as long as this isn't too intense. Then relax and release.

12. Pulse a few times on this side, then repeat on the other side.

Roll and Reach

Inspired by the Feldenkrais Method technique, this is a calming warm-up move for the whole body.

1. Lying on your back, bend the right knee and keep the other leg long.

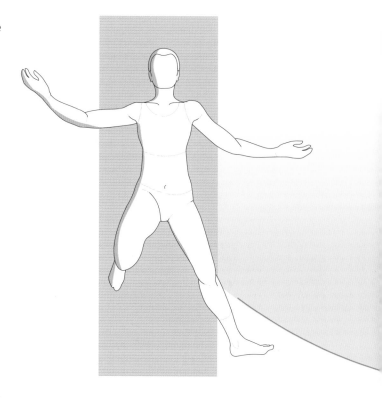

2. Take the left arm out to the side against the mat, about shoulder height.

3. Push into the right foot, notice how this makes the right hip and shoulder lift, then come back to the floor.

4. Keep repeating this pushing into the floor with the right foot, to create a rocking movement.

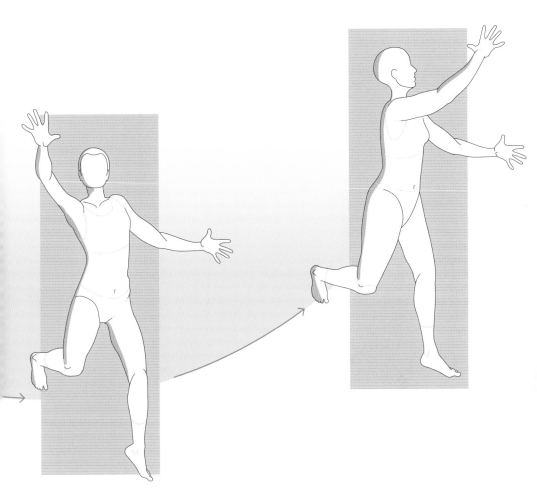

5. As you continue, you may want to push further, so that you can reach across your chest with your right arm and almost roll onto your left-hand side; then roll onto your back.

6. Use the right foot like a brake and accelerator to control the rocking and rolling motion: more pressure to roll, less pressure to come onto your back.

7. Repeat on the other side.

Rolling Over to Sit Up (and Back Down Again)

Sit Up

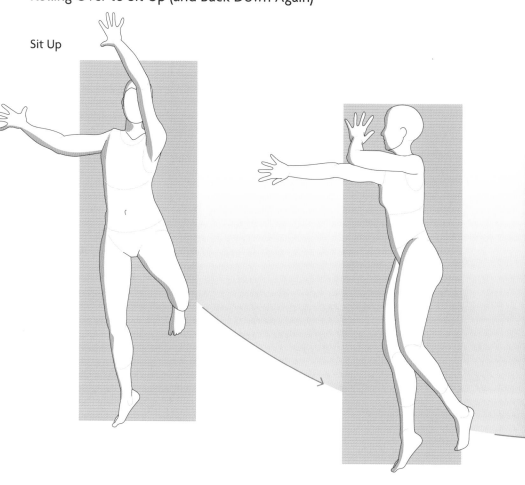

1. Lying on your back, bend the left knee and keep the other leg long.

2. Take the right arm out to the side against the mat, up by your right ear.

3. Push into the left foot, so the whole body rolls onto the right-hand side.

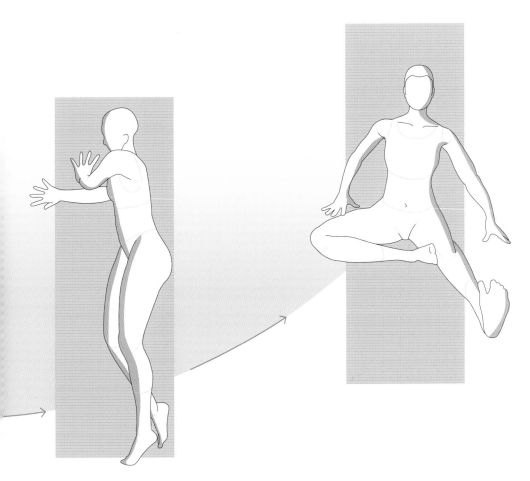

4. Bring the left hand in front of your face and push yourself up to sit.

5. As you come up, you'll notice that the left leg is straight and the right leg bent. This allows you to go straight into a Seated Head-to-Knee Pose (see page 176); alternatively, you could take the right leg behind you, into Half Pigeon (see page 190) or cross the right shin in front of the left, into Easy Pose (see page 170), and from there you can come up into standing.

Go Back Down

1. From Easy Pose (see page 170), straighten the left leg and extend the right arm to your side onto the mat, with the hand planted.

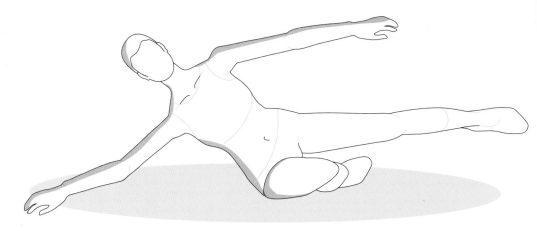

2. Follow the hand as you lower yourself back onto your right-hand side.

3. Start to take the left arm back across your chest, extending the arm to the left; this will begin to bring you onto your back.

4. At the same time, tuck in the legs and push into the outside edge of the right foot to bring the hips and legs back to centre.

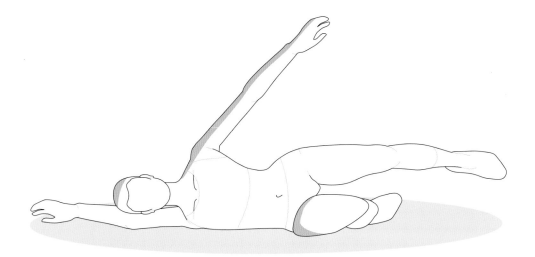

5. Push into the right foot, roll to the right and repeat on the other side.

6. See if you can repeat from side to side for a few rounds: take it slowly! The reversing of the steps on the way back down is challenging for the brain, but really good for creating new neural pathways.

Breath

The breath is central to the practice of yoga, whether it is physical or meditative. Yogis use the power of the breath to tap into the unconscious. At the same time, because breathing is also conscious, we can manipulate it to help us improve our health and wellbeing.

Many people do not breathe well. Several things can affect the quality of our breathing: muscle strength and flexibility, lung capacity, what's going on emotionally or in our minds, as well as illness and injury. Our stressful lives attack our unconscious breathing because it is so closely connected to the nervous system.

Physical yoga helps, because we have to breathe in order to move. Breathing while in the postures strengthens and lengthens our breathing capacity, while breathing when still makes us more aware of how we breathe. All physical yoga should include at least a few minutes of Breath Attention (see page 241), where you sit or lie down and simply focus on the mechanics of your breathing. This might include specific breathing techniques. When moving into or holding poses, keep breathing in a relaxed but controlled way that works for you.

There are many benefits to breathing well. It keeps our muscles relaxed and can relieve pain – especially the exhalation, which is related to the Parasympathetic Nervous System (see page 61). This then lowers the blood pressure and slows the heartbeat, leading to feelings of relaxation. Breathing well also helps with detoxification, because 70 per cent of toxins are released by breathing. The mechanics of breathing massages all our organs, via the diaphragm enhancing blood flow, and strengthens the heart and lungs. Good breath patterns release hormones known as endorphins, which have a pain-relief effect and balance the nervous system, including the Enteric Nervous System in the gut. This improves mood and the ability to manage our emotions and reactions. Conscious breath provides us with a readily accessible way to bring our focus to the inside, away from the busy mind, with various techniques that will be explored in this section.

The Anatomy of Breathing

Breathing is a wider process than simply what we feel in our chest. Our respiratory system includes the lungs, airways and muscles to enable breathing, while the circulatory system of the heart, veins, arteries and capillaries brings the blood to the lungs to allow for the exchange of oxygen and carbon dioxide.

There are two types of respiration: *external* via the lungs, where air enters from outside and then leaves roughly 12–15 times per minute; in someone with stress, this can be 20 times per minute. *Internal* respiration occurs at the cellular level, where cells and tissues are fed with oxygen, which is carried to the cells by blood and exchanged with carbon dioxide.

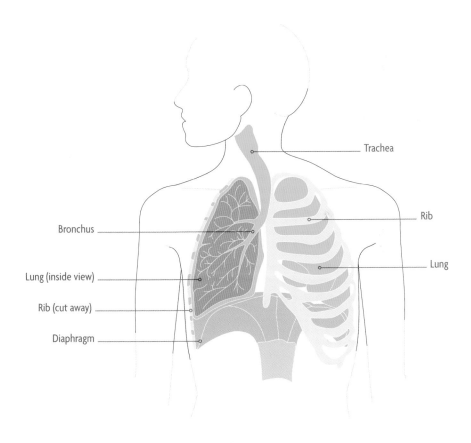

Trachea

Rib

Bronchus

Lung

Lung (inside view)

Rib (cut away)

Diaphragm

The thoracic cage contains the ribs, lungs and diaphragm. The lower back, or lumbar region, is affected by the movement of the diaphragm and abdominal walls, while the sacrum houses the pelvic wall and floor, and forms the bottom of the abdominal cavity. The shoulders are attached to the ribcage and spine, and movements of the arm and ribs will affect our breathing. Neck and cranial (skull) bones are also affected.

The Muscles of Breathing

There are many muscles involved in breathing, but the most famous is the thoracic diaphragm. This dome-shaped muscle separates the thoracic cavity from the abdomen, and sits attached to the lower ribs and spine. It is connected to the stomach and liver and other abdominal organs. The lungs sit on the diaphragm,

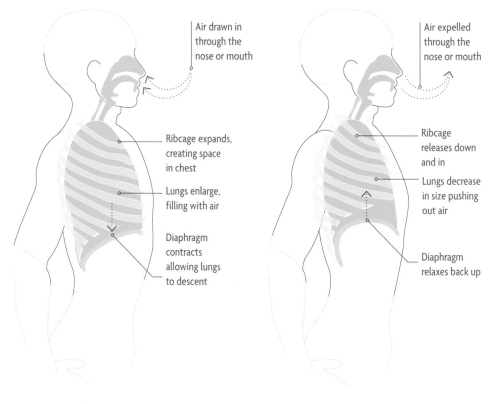

Air drawn in through the nose or mouth

Ribcage expands, creating space in chest

Lungs enlarge, filling with air

Diaphragm contracts allowing lungs to descent

Air expelled through the nose or mouth

Ribcage releases down and in

Lungs decrease in size pushing out air

Diaphragm relaxes back up

Inhale

Exhale

while the heart is on the central tendon of the diaphragm. Because of this set-up, every movement of the diaphragm – and so every breath – influences the organs that it lies in relation to.

The muscles around the back, ribs and shoulders are the secondary breathing muscles, and are needed to help lift the ribs away to allow the lungs to expand. The abdominal muscles are also secondary breathing muscles; they are needed to allow the diaphragm to return to its dome-shape after each exhale. The face, mouth and throat are also involved. Issues with any of these muscles can affect our breathing.

The Lungs

The lungs sit in the ribcage or thoracic cavity. The right lung is bigger than the left, to accommodate the shape of the heart on the left side. The lungs sit in their pleural membrane, which has two layers between them and the ribs. The lungs function by bringing oxygen into our system and releasing carbon dioxide – a waste product from our cells. The lungs have an elastic recoil, so when we inhale, they naturally get to a point where they allow us to breathe out. This recoil mechanism stimulates the diaphragm and other muscles to contract, to fully complete the exhale.

Breathing and the Nervous System

Breathing is an unusual bodily process, in that it is both unconscious and conscious. Sensors in the airways, brain, blood vessels, muscles and joints communicate to the respiratory system to make changes, to regulate the amount of oxygen. This will start an inhale; an exhale comes from the lungs' elastic recoil process. This breath process is unconscious and is controlled by the Autonomic Nervous System. When we are in a polluted city, we will breathe less to avoid taking in dirty particles; when exercising, we will breathe more.

The Parasympathetic Nervous System tells the diaphragm and muscles to move in response to the exchange of oxygen and carbon dioxide in the brain. The Sympathetic Nervous System actively increases the breathing rate through our stress response, such as exercise or the perception of a threat. This process releases norepinephrine, a chemical that increases the size of the bronchial tubes for breathing.

As the breath is so intrinsically linked to our nervous system and fascial network, even paying attention to the breath can be deeply uncomfortable for many people. If you have anxiety or suffer from panic attacks, please take care with all of the breathing exercises in this book.

WHAT HAPPENS WHEN WE BREATHE?

- The nervous system notes that more oxygen is needed in the brain.
- It sends a message to the diaphragm to move down, to allow the lungs to expand.
- The tummy and other organs move out of the way to make room for the diaphragm.
- The pelvis tilts slightly. The ribs expand. The shoulders and neck move slightly upward.

- At the top of the inhale, the lungs recoil to release the air.
- The diaphragm responds by contacting; the abdominal muscles contract to allow the diaphragm to return to its original shape.
- The pelvis tilts back, the shoulders and neck drop slightly, the ribs contract.
- All of this happens 17,000–30,000 times a day, usually without us even noticing!

Chest Breathing

Predominant use of the secondary breathing muscles rather than the diaphragm, known as "chest breathing", is a common cause of poor breathing. When this happens, the muscles of the shoulders and neck overwork and the abdominals are asleep. Many people breathe this way due to breathing through the mouth rather than the nose, poor posture and muscle tone, sitting for long periods and stress. Chest breathing impairs the diaphragm and puts a lot of stress on the lower back. The ribs find it hard to expand properly because the diaphragm has not moved out of the way, restricting the airflow. With this shallow breathing, it is hard to breathe air down into the bottom part of the lungs, which are also the widest, so stale air remains there. We then bring in less oxygen, which can make us feel sluggish.

When we breathe well, the entire body is moving. When we don't, the lack of movement can be destabilizing. The muscles and joints that we use to breathe are located in our trunk: these are also our core stabilizing muscles. When these are weak and immobile, our body will look to our extremities instead. Our nervous system will respond to this situation by compressing joints and tightening muscles in order to protect the body, causing more tension in the body and, ultimately, pain. This tension can further restrict breathing, causing an ongoing circle of issues.

Breathing in Postural Yoga

The ancient yogis discovered that playing with, and channelling, the breath could provoke altered states of consciousness – and that remains true for us today. We can practise *passive* breathing to induce a calm and relaxed state, and we can use *active* breath to stimulate the nervous system and ready the body for movement.

Many classes will start with some kind of passive breath awareness to calm the mind and bring attention inward. When done lying on the back, we feel supported, with a sense of safety. Breathing will then start to move into a more active phase as we prepare to move. Active breathing should ideally be done when you are at least sitting, so that there is muscular tension and the body begins to respond to slightly stressed conditions.

When we breathe in a conscious, active fashion, the diaphragm, abdominal wall and pelvic floor work to move air, but also to regulate air pressure in the abdominal cavity, which is key to core stability. The ability to breathe into the front, side and back of your abdominal cavity enables your hold torso to expand. This expansion signals to the brain that the spine is stable and is held.

The moment you hold your breath, breathe too hard or find it hard to breathe, you have taken the pose or movement too far. Holding the breath is a compensatory mechanism to help us find stability by bracing the core, and will happen when we lack real stability through the trunk. Holding the breath in this way stresses the nervous system. Remember to breathe through your nose as best you can throughout the whole yoga class as nasal breathing activates the diaphragm.

In more passive poses and styles of yoga, such as floor-based poses, yin yoga and restoratives, we can return to a more passive breath. This breath can still be aware: we can pay attention to it, perhaps visualize it or send it to places it would feel good to receive it.

Diaphragmatic Breathing

One of the first skills you may learn in a yoga class is how to move toward using the diaphragm for breathing. This is sometimes called the diaphragmatic breath, abdominal breathing or yogic breathing. The Tummy Breathing and Full Yogic Breath exercises on pages 238–239 show you how to activate the diaphragm.

Tummy Breathing

A simple way to start to bring the diaphragm into action is through
Tummy Breathing.

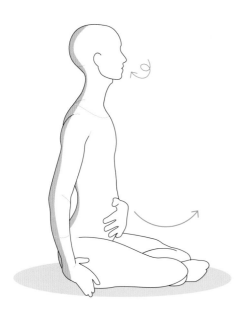
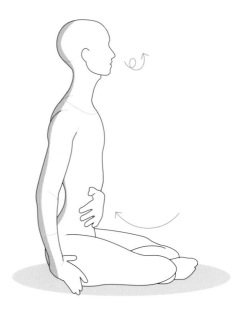

1. Sit up tall, with a long spine, on a chair or cushion. The lower back can be supported, but the torso should be free from constriction on all sides.

2. Bring the tongue to the roof of the mouth and breathe in and out through the nose. Allow the jaw to relax. Breathing through the nose activates the diaphragm.

3. Bring one hand onto the upper tummy, above the belly button. Breathe steadily and softly through the nose. Feel the tummy move against your hand as you breathe.

4. Breathe in your normal pattern for a few rounds.

5. Don't force the breath: visualize or sense it going into the space behind your hand (you are now actively drawing the breath into the lower and widest part of your lungs).

6. Repeat for a couple of minutes.

7. You might feel relaxed or sleepy, but avoid slouching: this breath activates the vagus nerve (see page 62), which runs past the diaphragm and switches on our rest-and-digest mode, the Parasympathetic Nervous System (see page 61).

Full Yogic Breath

A full yogic breath means fully activating the diaphragm, abdominal muscles and using all of your lung capacity.

1. Sit up with a long spine.

2. Start with Tummy Breathing (see opposite) in a steady, natural pattern through the nose.

3. Slightly slow down the breath, maybe 2–3 per cent.

4. As you breathe in, allow the tummy to expand away from the spine, creating room for the diaphragm to move down and the lungs to open.

5. Continue your inhale into the side of the ribcage, up under the armpits.

6. If comfortable, allow the inhale to continue into the upper chest, maybe slightly elevating the collarbones.

7. To exhale, follow the directions in reverse order: the upper chest exhales, ribs empty, belly sinks down to the spine, allowing the diaphragm to move up and "push" the remaining air out of the lungs.

8. The inhale and exhale should not be forced. It may take several rounds of breath, or even several practices, before you feel comfortable opening the upper chest.

9. Take your time and allow the breath to do its own work.

Conscious Breathing in Postures

Banana Breathing

1. Lying down with the legs extended and ankles wide, take your arms overhead.

2. Hold onto the right wrist with the left hand and take your arms, shoulders and torso over toward the left.

3. Cross your right ankle over your left, so that you make a banana shape on the floor.

4. Notice what happens to your breathing.

5. Can you send your breath more into the right-hand side of your torso, inflating the right lung and moving the muscles between the right side ribs?

6. Repeat on the other side, noting any differences.

Child's Breathing

1. Come into Child's Pose (see page 145), with the arms extended in front and the head supported on the floor or a block, knees apart.

2. Breathe into the belly and notice the movement of the tummy against the thighs. You might also feel the pelvis moving. Then notice the breath in the back of the body: from the sacrum up to the back of the ribs.

3. You can place one or both hands on the sacrum to feel the movement of the breath.

Lion's Breath

This can be done in the rounded-back Cat position (see page 144), Down Dog (see page 148) or Forward Fold (see page 98).

1. On the exhale, stick out the tongue and breathe out with a long "bleurgh" sound for the whole of the exhale.

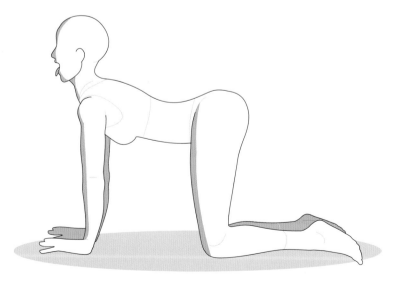

Breath Exercises

These exercises can be done lying or seated. You may wish to use a timer. Always breathe through the nose.

Simple Passive Breathing

1. With the eyes closed or soft, relax the jaw, tongue, throat and shoulders.

2. Bring your attention to your pattern of breath. There is no need to force or control your breathing.

3. Inhale: focus on feeling the nostrils expand and the sense of receiving the inhale into the body.

4. Exhale: gently release through the nose and feel the warm air on the upper lip.

5. Repeat for a minute or two, keeping your attention on the sense in the body of breathing.

Breath Attention

1. Bring one hand onto your navel and the other onto your chest.

2. Allow your breath to settle into its natural pattern and rhythm. Breathe through your nose.

3. Start to notice, with a curious, non-judgemental mind:
- Is the breath long, short or somewhere in the middle? Is the inhale different from the exhale?
- Is the breath deep or shallow, or in between?
- Is the breath jagged or smooth, or are the in-breath and out-breath different?
- Is each breath coming fast or slow? What is the frequency of the breath?
- Can you feel where the inhale starts in your body? Where does it stop?
  How about the exhale?
- Where do you most feel your breath? In the belly? The chest? The nostrils?

Ocean Breath or *Ujjayi* Breath

This is a subtle and soft breath practice.

1. Bring the tongue to the roof of the mouth to close the throat slightly.

2. Breathe in and out through the nose.

3. Feel the vibrations of the breath in the throat as well as the soft ocean sound. Avoid getting too strong and sounding like Darth Vader!

Three-Part Breath

1. Lying down, bend the knees, bring the hands to the lower belly and direct the breath here. Feel the belly and hands rise on the inhale and fall on the exhale. Repeat several times or for 1–2 minutes.

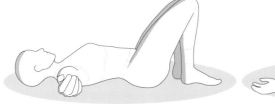 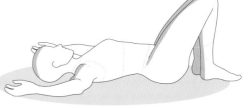

2. Take the arms out into a T shape and breathe into the ribs. Feel the ribcage expand outward on the inhale and contract on the exhale. Notice that the position of the arms helps to open the ribcage. Repeat as in step 1.

3. Take the arms overhead to the floor and breathe into the collarbones and armpits. Again the arm position helps find space in the upper chest.

4. Bring one hand to the belly and one hand to the chest: inhale, allowing the breath to fill the belly, ribs and collarbones; then exhale through the collarbones, ribs and belly. Repeat several times.

Further Breath Exercises

The following exercises are for those who feel comfortable working with the breath.

Extending the Exhale

1. Start with Tummy Breathing (see page 238), feeling the movement and engagement of the abdominals.

2. You can then use Ocean Breath (see opposite) but continue to feel the tummy move.

3. Take a few rounds and then count the average length of inhale and exhale: this is your starting point.

4. Whatever the count for both, lengthen the exhale by a count of one: e.g. inhale three, exhale four.

5. Repeat for several rounds, then see about lengthening the exhale by two counts: inhale three, exhale six. Repeat for a minute or so.

Counting the Breaths

1. Follow steps 1–3 of Extending the Exhale, until you have found your average breath count: the inhale and exhale are the same. Then extend both by a count of one, for three rounds.

2. Keep repeating up to a count of seven or eight (or maybe nine!). You will need to work on slowing down the breath and feeling it fill each section of the torso, in order to increase the count. It will take practice.

3. Once you have reached the longest count (without strain), go down a breath for one round, then down a breath again for the next, repeatedly, until you are back at your natural breath count, which might be around three or four.

Nine-Part Breath

This needs to be done sitting, so that you can access all the parts of the body used for breathing. At each stage, use an *ujjayi* breath (see page 242) to breathe into each part of the body. This practice creates awareness of where to breathe in poses, such as into the side of the ribs, in a twist. Some parts will be easier to breathe into than others: don't force anything; sometimes you just need to take your attention there.

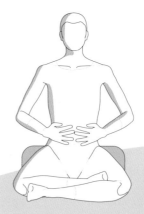

1. Hands on lower belly: allow the abdomen to rise and fall.

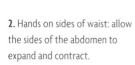

2. Hands on sides of waist: allow the sides of the abdomen to expand and contract.

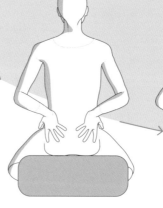

3. Hands on lower back: allow the back of the abdomen to move with the breath.

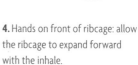

4. Hands on front of ribcage: allow the ribcage to expand forward with the inhale.

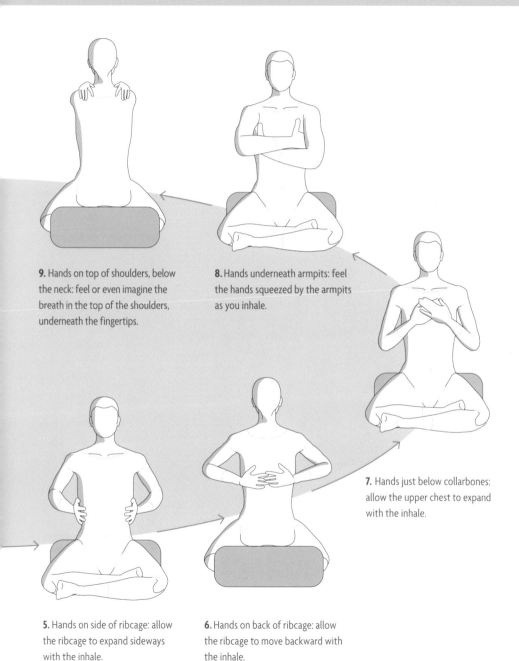

9. Hands on top of shoulders, below the neck: feel or even imagine the breath in the top of the shoulders, underneath the fingertips.

8. Hands underneath armpits: feel the hands squeezed by the armpits as you inhale.

7. Hands just below collarbones: allow the upper chest to expand with the inhale.

5. Hands on side of ribcage: allow the ribcage to expand sideways with the inhale.

6. Hands on back of ribcage: allow the ribcage to move backward with the inhale.

The Subtle Body

Even in the earliest yoga texts, the Upanishads, we saw references to a kind of internal body system and the movement of *prana*, or energy, with it. This system was widely developed during the Tantric period into a complete map of what is now known as the yogic, subtle or energy body.

It can be helpful to think of the subtle body in a couple of ways. First, when the system was conceptualized in the early medieval period, yogis were exploring their experience. Many centuries of practice had revealed commonalities, which were then described as energy moving in channels, winds moving through the body, and energy centres where certain emotions or states might be experienced. Second, modern physiology and neurology didn't exist, so this was possibly the only way to describe what was happening during meditation and breathwork and their aftermath. As we understand more about our bodies, energy and the mind, it is possible that one day we may have a 21st-century comprehension of the yogic subtle body.

Even if modern science fails to explain the subtle body definitively, don't let that diminish its importance. The subtle body contains important tools, which describe a possible experience that you may have, but they are not necessarily saying for certain that something is there. Conceptualizing the subtle body as a tool means that we don't need to believe in anything: let the model and the practices help you become more aware of, and better connected with, your emotions, moods and energy levels.

The *Nadis*

The subtle body is composed of a series of channels called *nadis* that flow through the body. Sources differ over how many there are, but most attention is given to the main three *nadis*: the *Susumna*, *Ida* and *Pingala*.

The *Susumna* runs from the crown of the head in front of the spine, in the very middle of the torso, down to the pelvic floor. Place one finger on the soft part of the crown and one finger on the perineum and notice whether you can sense a line of energy or awareness between these two points. The *chakras* are located along this line.

Also extending from the crown of the head to the pelvic floor are the *Ida* and *Pingala* *nadis*. These are sometimes shown as intertwining through each *chakra*, but can also be experienced just on the left side (*Ida*) and right side (*Pingala*).

Ida is said to represent "moon energy" and is therefore subtle, gentle, associated with white light and feelings of anxiety, grief and nervousness, but also compassion and creativity. *Pingala* is said to be the sun's energy and is associated with the colour red and with feelings of anger, guilt, irritation and resentment, but also drive and determination.

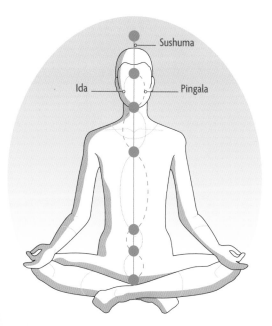

Ida — Sushuma — Pingala

Prana – the energy or life force – is said to flow through these *nadis* in the subtle body via winds called *vayus*. Yoga practices can be viewed as various ways to get *prana* into the body and moving wherever it is most helpful for us. This control of *prana* is called *pranayama*, or breath control, and involves various techniques using the breath, hand positions (*mudras*) and the management of locks inside the body (*bandhas*). We will look at these aspects of the subtle body in turn.

The *Chakras*

Chakras were a Tantric yoga innovation and are visualized meditative tools for practice, which are superimposed onto experiential energy centres that we all feel from time to time. If we look at our experiences as humans, they all have a somatic (bodily) component that is also experienced through the central channel: sexual desire; love and hate in the heart centre; drive and ambition in the solar plexus; choking up with emotion in the throat; concentration at the third eye on the forehead or a flash of insight.

The basis for the *chakras*, or energy centres, are these universal experiences, but it is important to remember they are tools, so a meditation might ask you to visualize a lotus-flower-shaped *chakra* at the heart to help with a practice, but that doesn't mean you have such a thing there, anatomically. Many people will also have energy-body experiences that do not match the major *chakra* points, and this is perfectly normal. When describing possible experiences, the idea is to see if it works for us, or not, at a particular time.

Many energy systems use the concept of *chakras*, but there are some differences between them. Some Indian systems use colours, such as red, white and gold, while others do not. The Western system, which is about 100 years old, also uses colours. This diversity is also reflected in how many *chakras* there are, and where they are located. Some systems have five, six, seven, twelve or twenty-one *chakras*; some have *chakras* in the legs.

The most well-known system has seven *chakras*, located as shown on the right. They are used with practices that are intended to achieve specific effects, to embody a particular emotion, for instance: to understand how one feels in the heart or the gut, and notice what is being held there, or is lacking; or to send gratitude or compassion into that area.

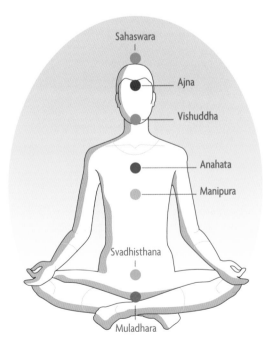

The Seven *Chakras*

Chakras are located along the central channel in the middle of the body, in front of the spine. This is where to take your awareness when practising, or you can visualize breathing into each area, as follows:

- **Sahaswara**: crown of the head – connection to the divine, to consciousness.
- **Ajna**: behind the eyes/mid-brain – intuition, insight and wisdom.
- **Vishuddha**: throat/centre of the throat – expression and truth.
- **Anahata**: heart, centre of the chest behind the breastbone – love, compassion, hate and heartbreak.
- **Manipura**: solar plexus – anger, power and drive.
- **Svadhisthana**: sacral, just below the belly button – desire, creativity, pleasure and enjoyment.
- **Muladhara**: perineum/pelvic floor – grounding and connection to the earth.

In the Tantric tradition *chakras* might be visualized as lotus flowers mapping Sanskrit syllables onto the energy body, with a seed mantra that is installed on the lotus petals. The seed mantras represent the elements, such as water and earth, and it is these that are installed in the *chakras* of the body to bring about certain effects.

When we do these practices, we are putting our intention into action. This signals to our subconscious that we are serious about this. If you spend half an hour a day doing a practice, your mind will start to register it, even if you can't see it. This allows your energetic body and nervous system to experience whatever you intend, even if you don't have it yet. This can be a very powerful and affirming experience.

When working with *chakras* it is advisable to start with simple visualization (mental image) techniques, to experience the embodiment of feeling. Installation of the elements is a sophisticated practice that requires a large degree of sensitivity and is not included here.

The *Koshas*

One aspect of the subtle body is the idea of each of us having layers – sheaths called *koshas*. In this model, a human being is described as having five sheaths that interpenetrate each other, encasing the soul like the layers of an onion. This model comes from the Taittiriya Upanishad, an ancient yoga text from c.600 BCE. As with many yogic technologies, this does not have to be taken literally: the *koshas* are a model that can be used to fine-tune our awareness.

The *koshas* can refine our awareness of who we are – both in this life and more metaphysically. Most of us have the first layer, *Annamaya Kosha* – the gross or physical body – available to us. We might not be fully aware of its nuances, but we will know when something hurts or we feel ill or hungry. We are also well aware of our mental sheath, *Manomaya Kosha*: all the thoughts, images and stories that pass through our minds.

The *koshas* show us that we can become deeply embodied and can create space around thoughts and stories. In addition, connecting to our energy *kosha*, *Pranamaya Kosha*, allows us to tap into our own vitality and that of nature; we become better at managing our energy in different circumstances and at understanding our needs. As we get better at dropping into *Vijnanamaya Kosha*, we can learn to listen to our intuition, rather than simply relying on the thinking mind. And finally we can find our way to *Anandamaya Kosha* – the bliss that lies at the heart of our existence. We can actually become aware of all the sheaths or *koshas* simultaneously and have an expanded sense of ourselves.

The *koshas* are seen as intertwined layers that are part of us, and understanding these sheaths enables us to get to know ourselves.

The Five *Koshas*

- *Annamaya Kosha*, **the physical body**: learning to be in our physical body, not thinking about, not disassociated from it; an awareness of different body parts, organs, movement; moving with an awareness of the body.
- *Pranamaya Kosha*, **the energetic body**: feeling energized or listless; feeling energy around the heart or head; noticing the energy of other people, or of places and food.
- *Manomaya Kosha*, **the mental layer**: thoughts, images, fantasies, daydreams; also the powerful mental structures formed by the beliefs, opinions and assumptions that we have absorbed from our families and culture, as well as from our accumulated mental patterns.

- *Vijnanamaya Kosha,* **the wisdom layer**: the sense of inner knowing, intuition, insight; often used in writing, painting, composing and other creative works.
- *Anandamaya Kosha,* **the bliss layer**: the most hidden part of us, yet its subtle presence is felt as the instinctive sense that life is worth living: that to be alive is good.

Understanding the *koshas* helps us to get to know ourselves. Underneath these layers is said to be Atman, the true self: beyond the mind, beyond the physical body, beyond knowledge.

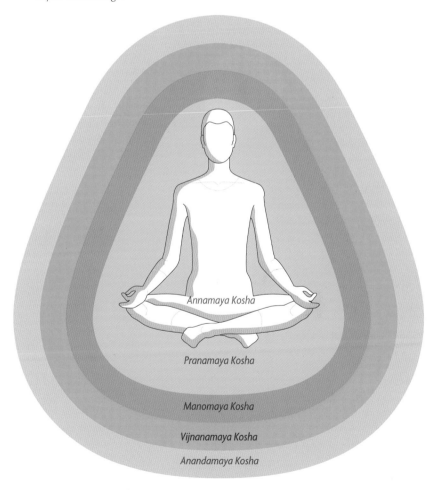

Annamaya Kosha

Pranamaya Kosha

Manomaya Kosha

Vijnanamaya Kosha

Anandamaya Kosha

Pranayama

Pranayama means the control of prana using the breath, and is first referenced as a practice in the early Upanishads. It originated with the Sramana movement c.500 BCE, and this makes it one of the oldest yoga techniques available to us. Pranayama practices have remained fairly similar to those first revealed in the early texts although there are more modern forms such as Wim Hof and Buteyko breathing. These both bring a change to the nervous system and affect the energy body through controlled breathing and breath holds.

As we have seen, day-to-day breathing is an automatic, unconscious process, governed by the Autonomic Nervous System (see page 61). Pranayama moves the breath into a controllable state using the neocortex, so it is not "just breathing". Without the ability to breathe well, however, pranayama will be difficult.

Pranayama techniques, both ancient and modern, may have an element of force about them. Students should take care with this and acknowledge whether force is what they really need, or if more subtle visualization practices or gentle breathing techniques might be more beneficial. The key is in understanding what you need at a particular time.

The Five Winds Or Vayus

Pranayama exercises are designed to move prana around the body in certain directions for specific purposes. The winds are seen as directions for prana to move through the nadis, and our subtle-body practices work with these winds: using visualization, bandhas and mudras and pranayama techniques themselves.
- **Prana Vayu**: works to bring prana into the body, on the inhale.
- **Apana Vayu**: works to release "stuff" from the body, on the exhale.
- **Samana Vayu**: works with the belly and solar plexus to generate fire and energy.
- **Vyana Vayu**: works to circulate prana throughout the body.
- **Udana Vayu**: works to move prana upward.

Pranayama Exercises

As pranayama works as one foot in the physical world and one foot in meditation, it is great for calming the mind and preparing for a seated meditation, or it can be done on its own. The focus and control of the breath work with the concept of pratyahara, or withdrawal of the senses. Pranayama exercises need to be done sitting upright on a cushion on a chair, with a long spine.

Intentional Breath

A simple *pranayama* for bringing the attention to our breathing and making it more conscious and deliberate. Keep the mouth and lips soft when you breathe out.

- Inhale nose.
- Exhale mouth.
- Inhale nose.
- Exhale nose.
- Repeat for 20 rounds.

Ratio Breathing

This improves our breath control so that we can manage *prana*. It is sometimes called Square Breathing and can involve breath retention, so if this makes you feel anxious or uncomfortable, skip the retention, focus on the slight pause and stay with the counted breathing instead. A typical starting ratio breath would be:

- Inhale for a count of four.
- Pause with the breath retained for a count of two.
- Exhale for a count of four.
- Pause with the breath held out for a count of two.

You can change the ratio to whatever works with your length of breath – for example 6:3 up to 12:6! Do not force your length of breath; you may want to spend some time practising the Counting the Breaths exercise (see page 243) to increase the length of the breath before you attempt Ratio Breathing.

Shining Skull Breath (*Kapalabhati*)

This *pranayama* was considered a cleansing practice in the Hathapradipika yoga treatise, and is often taught in group classes. Also known as the Pumping or Skull Cleansing Breath, it forces *prana* upward and is similar to Wim Hof breathing. Take it easy, by reducing the breath count, if you have anxiety or feel ungrounded.

Preparation

1. Blow your nose, if needed.
2. *Kapalabhati* "pumping" comes from the lower abdominals, not the tummy.
3. Sit and let your lower belly relax completely, then on the next exhale draw the lower belly in slightly.
4. As you inhale, again completely relax the lower belly, allowing it to get big.
5. You can have a hand on the belly, if it helps to feel this.

Practice

1. Exhale fully and draw in the belly, then simply relax the lower abdominals with a passive inhale.
2. To "pump", draw the belly in, to push the air out of the lungs, quite forcibly, then fully relax the belly again with a passive inhale. This happens quite quickly. Then pump again and repeat.
3. After 20 pumps, draw the belly in to exhale to empty.
4. Inhale long and slow as much as you can, then exhale long and slow, as if a thread is being pulled out of your nose.
5. After this exhale, simply release the belly with a passive inhale and relax – watch the breath: do you actively need to breathe? If you do, notice the quality of the breath. It might be very shallow and slight. This is due to the blood being very oxygenized. Simply pay attention to the breath and sit until your breathing returns to normal and the mind becomes distracted.
6. Repeat two more times.

Alternate Nostril Breathing (*Nadi Shodhana*)

Alternate nostril breathing focuses the mind by switching the breath through each side of the nose; you can add a count to the breath, for added concentration. This breath is balancing *prana* in both the *Ida* and *Pingala nadis* (see page 247), and is good for concentration and relaxed alertness. Avoid it if you have a cold or a blocked nose Use your predominant hand and close the first and second fingers to the palm, leaving the thumb, ring and little fingers lifted. If right-handed, use your thumb to close the right nostril, and the ring finger to close the left. Keep eyes closed, or at least very soft and relaxed.

Preparation

1. Start by closing the left nostril, and breathe in and out through the right. Then close the right and breathe in and out through the left.

Practice

1. Close the left nostril, and breathe in through the right.
2. Close the right nostril, and exhale through the left.
3. Inhale through the left.
4. Close the left and exhale right.
5. This is one round. You can repeat for 10–20 rounds.

For added focus, you can count each inhale/exhale. For example, inhale for a count of four, exhale for a count of four. When you have finished your rounds, pause with the eyes still closed and return to your natural breathing for a minute or so.

Eight Classical Breaths

The Hathapradipika included Eight Classical Breaths, some of which are taught in classes today (except for numbers 6 and 7 below).

1. **Bhastrika or the Bellow Breath**: this advanced breath technique is cleansing and invigorating; it pushes *prana* up, using short inhales and exhales through the nose like a bellows or pump, with a strong contraction of the diaphragm. There can be a dizzy or high feeling. Be careful with anxiety.

2. **Ujjayi or Ocean Breath**: this can bring feelings of being uplifted and of success, as it raises *prana* (see page 242 for how to do it).

3. **Sitkari**: a cooling breath, whereby the teeth are close together, but the lips are open. Inhale through the mouth so that the air travels over the wet teeth, and exhale through the nose.

4. **Sitali**: another cooling breath, which requires the tongue to be rolled with the outside edges in, like a straw. Inhale through the tongue and exhale through the nostrils.

5. **Brahmari or Buzzing Bee Breath**: this involves closing the ears with the hands and humming through the lips like a buzzing bee and really brings the attention inward. It can be practised in Child's Pose (see page 145) for an introspective experience.

6. **Mucha**: a long inhale retention with the throat lock *Jalahandabandha* until fainting.

7. **Plavini**: a holding breath in the stomach and chest, long enough until the body feels as if it is floating.

8. **Surya Bhedhana**: right nostril breathing – breathe in through the right nostril and exhale through the left. This is said to stimulate the *Pingala nadi* on the right-hand side, which can be a stimulating and enlivening practice.

Mudras and Bhandas

Mudras and bandhas are techniques used to manage energy in the yogic body. Mudras are hand gestures and seals, and bandhas are internal contractions or locks inside the body. These are subtle techniques that can be added to asanas, pranayama or meditation practices.

Mudras

Different hand positions are said to affect different aspects of the brain and nervous system, and therefore energy or prana. Here are five common mudras that can be used in your practice:

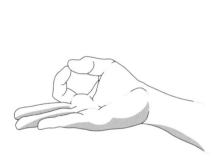

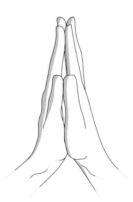

- **Chin or Jnana Mudra**: said to help connect us to a more fundamental state. To do it: bring the thumb and first finger to touch, with the other fingers open but relaxed. Place the hands in this mudra palm-down on the knees for a more grounded feeling, or palm-up to feel more receptive.

- *Anjali Mudra:* shows respect to oneself and to others; used in traditional greetings and also at the end of classes. To do it: simply bring the hands together at the base of the heart, fingers pointing upward.

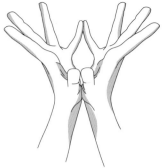

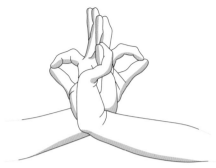

- **Lotus or *Padma Mudra***: the lotus flower floating on the water is said to represent our ability to rise above fear and attachment. To do it: start with the hands together; spread open the hands and fingers, keeping the base of the hands, thumbs and little fingers together. The middle fingers stay open. Nestle the thumbs into the breastbone.

- **Fearless Heart Mudra**: this can be used to help keep the heart open, even during difficult times; it is good to use with heart meditations. To do it: bring the hands into *Anjali Mudra*, then cross the right wrist in front of the left, so the backs of the hand are facing each other. Hook the first, second and little fingers together, right over left. Then touch the open ring fingers to the thumbs.

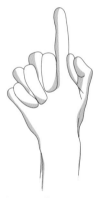

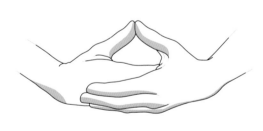

- *Kali Mudra*: find your inner strength and fearlessness with the goddess Kali. To do it: bring the hands, together then interlace the fingers except the index fingers, which point forward. You can rest the inside of the wrists against the solar plexus.

- **Meditation or *Dhyana Mudra***: provides calming energy for meditation. To do it: place your hands on your lap, left palm underneath, palms facing up, with the tips of the thumbs touching.

Bandhas

Bandhas are subtle muscle contractions in specific areas; they are an advanced practice used in meditation, pranayama and asanas. When in a pose, follow the directions to engage and integrate the muscles and joints for stability, then maybe gently add the bandhas if you are interested in exploring the control of prana.

Bandhas are generally used with pranayama and often involve retention of the breath, known as kumbhaka. Retaining the breath in or out is an advanced practice and is not used in this book. If you wish to explore it further, find a teacher experienced in pranayama and bandha techniques.

For all the bandhas the engagement of muscles in the lock is subtle; aim for about 50 per cent of your maximum. If you pull in too hard, the body can go into fight-or-flight response, which is not helpful in your practice.

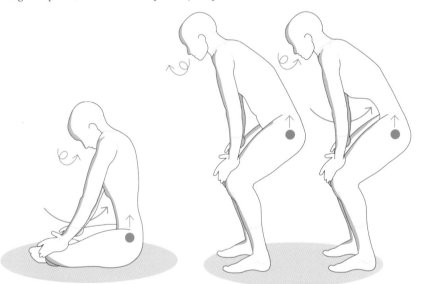

- *Jalandhara Bandha*, the throat lock: Engage by slightly bringing the chin down to close the throat. This is used in breath retention on the inhale.

- *Uddiyana Bandha*, the abdominal lock: Strongly exhale, relax the abdominals, but let the chest inflate; you can then engage the abdominal muscles to pull the belly in and up.

- *Mula Bandha,* the root lock at the pelvic floor: Gently draw up the pelvic floor as if you are preventing yourself from urinating. There should not be too much squeeze: if the buttocks engage, then you have gone too far.

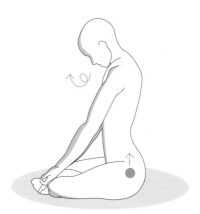

Standing Breath of Fire

It is really good to get rid of anything stagnant, especially after a frustrating day! Do this on an empty stomach!

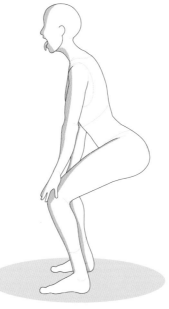

1. Stand with feet apart, knees bent and a sense of buoyancy: make sure you can bend the knees and come forward comfortably to place the hands on the thighs, with the back slightly rounded.

2. Inhale fully, then do a short, quick exhale as if pushing all the air out of the lungs, drawing the abdominals in to help move the air out.

3. Relax the abdominal muscles, then allow the thoracic cavity (ribs and chest) to expand without inhaling.

4. Then actively lift draw up the abdominals toward the spine.

5. Drop the chin into *Jalandhara Bandha* at the same time.

6. Relax, breathe in and stand up when ready: do not hold for too long.

Meditation

Meditation has become increasingly popular over the past ten years or so, with a proliferation of apps and courses that you can use for practice. The choice of which type of meditation to practise will depend on the individual and what they need at that moment. Meditation also has some contraindications, especially for mental-health conditions, and we will review this below.

Traditionally, starting with the *Sramana* movement and via classical yoga, meditation is seen as control of the mind. Attention is brought inward, away from daily distractions and stimuli; this is known as *pratyahara*, and involves more concentrative meditation techniques. Control of the mind involves improved focus and attention, increased concentration and calming the fluctuations of the mind.

Focus and attention are two of the main aspects of meditation, which the corporate world has now latched onto, although this is really only the beginning. Concentration is needed to allow the mind to focus on whatever the meditation technique or practice is: following the breath, watching a candle or visualizing. Once the mind has quieted, our brain switches to alpha waves (see page 67) and it is possible to access a deeper layer: the subconscious. There are many uses for this practice, especially in creative endeavours, and in therapy and healing. Allowing what is beneath the thinking, analytical part of our mind to emerge can bring forth answers and ideas that we might never otherwise hear. It can also enable a deep sense of relaxation and release.

Accessing these other states of consciousness has long been part of the practice and goal of yoga. Some of these altered states bring a sense of expansion: connecting to hidden parts of ourselves and our psyches or, further still, accessing a sense of awareness and pure consciousness. Many of us will only ever experience this in small glimpses or in moments, although long-term practice can bring about this state for longer.

For the everyday practitioner, extended periods in altered states are not necessary. However, the ability to access a different state to the one you habitually find yourself in is a key life skill, as is the ability to develop a different relationship with the thinking mind. Most of us will never "stop thinking", but that isn't really the goal. It is how best to create space around our thoughts, so that they become tools for us to use when needed, and less troublesome for us when we are agitated and fluctuating. Can we find ways to access the space behind the thinking mind, where deeper layers of understanding and intuition lie, and which may offer greater healing, more rest and connection and different perspectives from the constant chatter in our heads?

As with physical yoga, meditation has been sold as a relaxation aid or an answer to stress and anxiety. While these benefits can be seen by some practitioners, they are not guaranteed. There is considerable ongoing research into the negative effects of meditation, and some practitioners report that practising it can make them feel more anxious, or numb and disassociated. Research is also ongoing into the link between some forms of meditation and anxiety, depression, disassociation and even psychosis.

If you feel worsening anxiety, depression and lack of connection from your meditation practice, stop and consult your doctor. Not all practices are suitable for everyone.

Mindfulness

Mindfulness is a concept developed by the Buddha and is the practice of paying attention to the present moment, on purpose and without judgement. It has become very popular as a modern technique, although now it is often presented as separate from its spiritual home.

Mindfulness meditation practices are a specific style of meditation designed to cultivate the ability to pay attention to whatever arises: sounds, breath, sensations, moods, thoughts and feelings. Additional practices include paying attention while walking, mindful drawing and colouring. Mindfulness is a key skill to cultivate during physical yoga practice in order to pay attention to the breath and the body.

Mantras

Mantras are groups of words or syllables in Sanskrit, which, if infused with *prana*, are said to generate an emotional response in the listener. They originate from both the Vedic and Tantric traditions, although the only commonality is the chant Om. Mantras are used in Tantric meditations combined with visualizations to install the elements, such as water or fire, or other attributes into the person chanting.

Traditionally you cannot choose a mantra from a book. It is either transmitted through a teacher or you can notice if you have an emotional response to it, upon hearing it. Even listening on a device can be enough, if the mantra is alive with *prana* and generates a response in you. This is due to the effect of *prana*, but also to the impact of sound vibrations throughout your body as you listen or chant.

Mantras can be used in meditation as a practice to focus the mind and allow the sound vibration and *prana* to move through you as you sit. In this book any suggested mantra is used for this purpose, but you can research online recordings.

Some teachers will talk of profound experiences, deep devotion or a sense of connection from well-known mantras, such as *Om Namah Shivaya*. This means "Adoration to Lord Siva", where each syllable represents an element, such as earth, and overall infers that "universal consciousness is one". If you are interested in mantras, then listening to recordings online to find one that resonates with you is an easy place to start.

Preparing for Meditation

It can help to do some preliminary yoga poses, mindful movement and breathwork prior to sitting. These exercises enable the nervous system to calm, so that as you enter meditation you are less physically and mentally agitated. Meditation requires a quiet space away from distractions, where you feel safe, as you are about to close your eyes and go inward. You can sit on a chair or on a cushion on the floor, but the spine must be long and ideally self-supporting. If sitting on a chair, ensure the feet are flat on the floor and the lower back is supported. Remember: you are not going into deep relaxation; you are looking for a pose that is a state of relaxed alertness – a mix of effort (*sthira*) and ease (*sukha*).

You might use an app or guided meditation, or set a timer with intermittent chimes to keep you present and let you know when the time is up. You may also want a blanket, warm socks or a sweater, as the body temperature can drop. It is usually advisable to develop a routine around meditation: a set time every day when you do it. If you meditate before bed, that's okay, but not lying in bed, as you are likely to fall asleep.

Different Types of Meditation

There are many kinds of meditation, from numerous traditions, so it can be helpful to understand them and what they might be used for. Many types of meditation are Buddhist, while others come from other Indian spiritual traditions, such as Vedanta and Saiva Tantra. More modern forms of meditation, such as mindfulness, are based on older practices, often with the spiritual element removed.

Concentration

Concentration involves focusing on one object, while allowing everything else to fade into the background. The object of meditation can be outside the body, such as a candle flame, or inside it, such as the breath or a mantra. A more subtle version would be to focus on energy centres in the body.

The most simple job we can give ourselves is to "watch the breath": we might need to count the breath softly to ourselves, or gently say, "Breathing in, breathing out", to really focus the mind on its job. The benefits of this are that the breath is available everywhere at any time. Even in a meeting or on the bus, we can simply pay attention to our breathing, without needing an app or a guide.

Certain Tantric meditations used the idea of entrainment, which provides several jobs for the mind to do. Not only does this occupy the mind but the "jobs" have specific intentions, such as drawing attention to the heart.

Awareness

Awareness incorporates mindfulness practices such as mindful eating or walking; sitting with awareness of the breath; or with awareness of being aware. It may often have an element of self-inquiry. Mindfulness means paying attention to what is arising in any given moment – breath, sounds, feelings, thoughts – allowing them to come into awareness and then pass away again. This cultivation of watching and noticing is known in some schools as *Vipassana* and is an advanced practice. It is difficult to sit and pay attention without the mind wandering; and it can be quite dissociative or ungrounding for some people.

Integrative Meditation

This involves switching from placing attention on an object and being with whatever arises. Many modern mindfulness meditations are based on this technique, where the attention switches from what is coming up, back to the breath. Tantric meditations can also involve switching from visualization to awareness. With considerable practice, this absorption can lead to *samadhi* (meditative consciousness).

Yoga Nidra

This is a popular guided meditation, which can be done lying down, where you are taken through different states of consciousness and then back to awakeness. It is also known as Yogic Sleep and is deeply restorative.

Other kinds of meditation include contemplation, such as on a word or some text; self-talk processes; and visualizations such as "going on a journey".

3
HOW TO LIVE YOUR YOGA

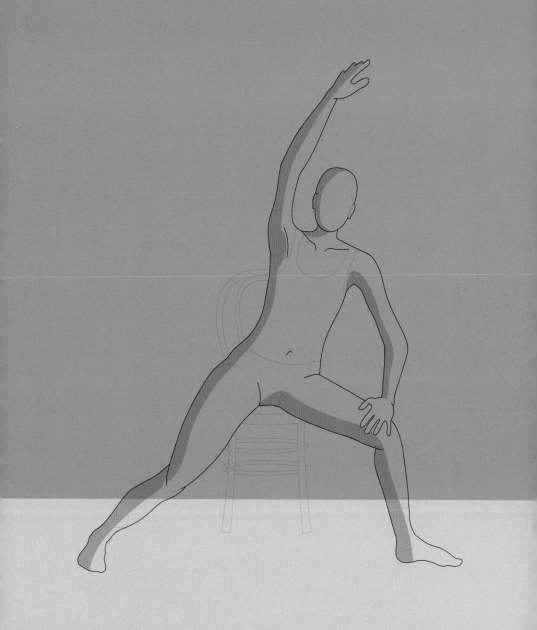

How to Practise

There are a variety of practices in this part of the book, which are not prescriptive or exhaustive – they are simply ideas to get you started. Make sure you have enough space for your mat, props and to roll around in. You might choose some music or light a candle. See if you can be undisturbed for the duration of your practice.

Dynamic Practices

- You can repeat the mini-flows once, twice or more. The more you repeat them, the more you may find the body remembers the poses and movements, and the less you need to think about them or refer to the book. This enables you to be in your body and to have your own experience.
- Once you have moved a little in the pose, pause, find stillness and breathe. This allows the nervous system to take an imprint of what you are doing, and provides a moment to *feel*.
- Move slowly, as if the room is full of thick, dark treacle. You are moving slowly enough that the breath is calm and smooth and you can feel every muscle, engagement and area of space that you are investigating.
- Explore and experiment: you can move your arms differently. You could take a different version of a pose, add in a new pose or leave one out. Use blocks or a chair to find more space.
- Don't skip *Savasana* (see page 206)! It's really tempting when you're at home on your own – but it is the most important part of the practice.

Yin/Restorative Practice

- Set a timer for 2–3-minute intervals, so that you know when to change pose or side, without constantly having to check your watch.
- Spend time getting set up in each pose and ensuring that you are fully supported.
- Find the soft side of your edge: about 60 per cent of your range of movement (see page 47), or use props so that you can relax completely without tension.
- Once in a pose, be as still as you can, unless you want to move out of it.
- Come out as slowly as you went in: do a counterpose or find gentle movements, before moving on.
- If you are hypermobile, use all the props to make the poses restorative rather than stretchy: your body should feel completely supported in all the positions.
- Caution: Do not do a yin practice if you are pregnant, as the effect of the relaxin hormone released during pregnancy, and long holds, can be unhelpful for the connective tissue.
- Don't skip *Savasana*!

Meditation and Breathing Practices

- Find a quiet space where you won't be disturbed.
- Use a timer.
- Sit on a chair or cushion that allows your spine to be long: you can lean back, but avoid slouching.

Practice in Everyday Life

In addition to scheduled practice time, this book also includes various suggestions for how to bring in practice throughout the day. By practice, we mean cultivating awareness, and bringing attention to the body, mind and emotions. This is the essence of yoga practice and can involve noticing when you need to stand up and move, when you need to sit and be quiet, or process emotion or practise noticing more of the smaller things in life that light you up. Being able to bring practice this way can be transformative as it becomes a way of life rather than another thing on the to-do list.

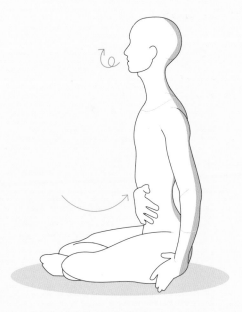

Tummy Breathing

A Practice to Energize and Wake Up

This practice will gently stimulate the nervous system so that we move into the social side of the vagus nerve (see page 62). Pay attention to how you feel throughout the practice and notice any impact on your energy levels.

Opening

- In Easy Pose (see page 170), Breath Attention or Simple Passive Breathing (see page 241) (1–2 minutes).
- Ocean Breath (see page 242) (1–2 minutes).
- Wake up the face and jaw by moving the tongue, jaw and brow.
- Gently turn the head from side to side; roll the chin along the collarbones and up to the ceiling.

Preparation

- Seated Cow/Cat (see page 172), then circular Seated Cow/Cat, going in both directions.
- Seated Side Bend (see page 173) with Rib Massaging (see page 186) x 3 on both sides. Find somewhere to pause on both sides and breathe.

Transition and Warm-Up

- Advanced Cow/Cat (see page 220) x 3, end on your belly and rest.
- Wide-Armed Cobra (see page 154), waving up and down, x 3.
- Push back to Child's Pose (see page 145).
- Low Lunge with right foot forward (see page 104).
- Low-Lunging Cow/Cat (see page 106).
- Swing the ankle inward, turn to the left and find Side Plank A (see page 134).
- 3 x Non-Linear Arm Circles (see page 59) then pause where it feels interesting and breathe for a moment.
- Top hand to the floor, move through All Fours (see page 138) to Child's Pose. Rest and focus on the breath for a moment.
- Repeat on the other side.

Dynamic Standing Poses

- Down Dog (see page 148), pedalling the legs and moving the hips.
- Walk forward to Forward Fold (see page 98) and roll up to stand.
- Chair Pose to Hunchback (see page 129).
- High Lunge with right leg back (see page 107) to High-Lunging Cow/Cat (see page 110) x 3.
- Drop the back heel in and lengthen both legs for Reverse Triangle (see page 122).
- Push off the front foot and turn to Horse Pose (see page 123), squatting and straightening the legs.
- Turn the left foot in, right toes forward, find Warrior 2 (see page 100) facing the other direction.
- Reach the left hand forward and step to Tree Pose (see page 111). Pause then explore Twisted Tree (see page 112).
- Reach up to the ceiling, transition through Forward Fold to Down Dog and choose a *Vinyasa* option (see page 220).
- You can repeat on the same side or alternate side as many rounds as feels suitable.

Closing

- Thoracic Twist (see page 79).
- Supported Bridge (see page 169).

Pranayama and *Savasana*

- Alternate Nostril Breathing (see page 254).
- Choose a *Savasana* option (see page 206).

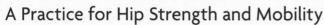

A Practice for Hip Strength and Mobility

In this practice we work with the feeling of engaging, rather than purely stretching. This engagement comes from the connection to the floor, so there is a strong foot-to-hip relationship. Always stay within your active range of motion.

Opening
- Start lying down. Breath Attention or Simple Passive Breathing (see page 241) (1–2 minutes).
- Ocean Breath (see page 242) (1–2 minutes).
- Wake up the face and jaw by moving the tongue, jaw and brow, then turn the head from side to side.

Preparation
- Active Knees-to-Chest Pose with single knee (see page 199), circle the knee.
- Active Sleeping Pigeon (see page 191) – knees can come toward the chest to make hip circles, but don't use your hands! Repeat on the other side.
- All Fours Hip Circles (see page 139).
- Cow/Cat (see page 144) or Advanced Cow/Cat (see page 220) x 2–3 rounds.
- Rest in Child's Pose (see page 145).

Transition and Warm-Up
- Rolling Lunge with right leg outside the right hand (see page 92).
- Elastic Lunge (see page 106).
- Wide-leg stance, shifting to Surfer (see page 127) with hands on the floor and pulse, feeling the foot-to-hip connection; then repeat on the other side.
- Step back to Down Dog (see page 148), then Advanced Cow Cat.
- From All Fours (see page 138), step the right leg out to the side and bring the left hand under the left shoulder for Side Plank A (see page 134). Find the sense of drawing into the pelvis: lift the right leg and pulse a little here.
- Step the lifted foot behind you flat onto the floor, knee bent with open hips for Popstar (see page 162).

- Sit down, then lie down to rest.
- Repeat, starting with left leg coming forward for Rolling Lunge.

Dynamic Standing Poses
- Down Dog.
- Walk hands back to feet, Squat (see page 130), play with Half Squat (see page 131).
- Heels drop, knees bend, roll up to stand.
- Warrior 2 with right leg back (see page 100).
- Rainbow Warrior (see page 103), push down through both feet, find the engagement through the feet, legs, pelvis and tummy, lift both arms.
- With front knee bent, Half Moon Pose (see page 116).
- Let the top leg come to the floor and push up to Reverse Triangle (see page 122), lifting the chest toward the ceiling, take one or two breaths.
- Turn front toes in, Wide-Legged Forward Fold (see page 99).
- Wide-leg Rolling *Vinyasa* (see page 222).
- Repeat sequence 2–3 times on one side, starting with Squat and then the other side.

Closing
- Half Lord-of-the-Fishes Pose (see page 177.)
- Wide-Arm Back Extension (see page 80).
- Supported Bridge (see page 169) or Supported Shoulder Stand (see page 193).

Pranayama and *Savasana*
- Ocean Breath (2–3 minutes).
- Choose a *Savasana* option (see page 206) .

A Practice for Resilience and Strength

This is a strong practice, using the mid-back and glutes. The core is engaged through this relationship with the pelvis and upper torso. Move at your own pace and take all the pauses for rest!

Opening

- Start seated. Feel the breath in the belly and ribs, front and back (1–2 minutes).

Preparation

- All Fours exploration: Cow/Cat (see page 144), Hip and Rib Circles (see page 139).
- Advanced Cow/Cat (see page 220).
- Kneeling Cow-Faced Shoulder Opener (see page 182).

Transition and Warm-Up

- Seated Head-to-Knee Pose with left knee bent and right leg straight (see page 176), checking in with the jaw and neck.
- Seated Side Bend to left (see page 173), then reach to right ankle with left hand x 3.
- Pause in the next Seated Side Bend and breathe.
- Popstar with right foot forward, left hand behind (see page 162).
- Strong through hand and foot to lift other foot to turn over to Tiger Plank (see page 137) (30 seconds).
- Rest in Child's Pose (see page 145), if needed.
- Down Dog (see page 148) to Three-Legged Dog lifting right leg (see page 150), then take knee to nose x 3.
- Step to Low Lunge (see page 104). Pause and breathe here.
- Lift back knee, shift to Surfer (see page 127), pulse a little, then move back to Low Lunge x 3. Hands might come away from the floor.
- Advanced Cow/Cat or Rolling *Vinyasa* (see page 222).
- Down Dog to Side Dog (see page 153).
- Spiral round to sit and pause.
- Repeat on the other side.

Dynamic Standing Poses

- Seated Head-to-Knee Pose with left knee bent and right leg straight, checking in with the jaw and neck.
- Popstar with right foot forward, left hand behind.
- Strong through hand and foot to lift other foot to turn over to Forward Fold (see page 98).
- Speed Skater (see page 89) to Standing Splits (see page 115) x 3.
- Forward Fold and roll up to stand.
- Pause and breathe. Get used to standing upright.
- Chair Pose (see page 128).
- Step back to High Lunge (see page 107).
- High Lunge to Winged Lunge (see page 109), then Surfer to High Lunge x 3.
- Down Dog to Advanced Cow/Cat or Rolling *Vinyasa*.
- Option to pause in Child's Pose.
- Down Dog to Three-Legged Dog, lifting right leg, then bringing lifted leg underneath to sit.
- Repeat on the other side.

Closing

- Basic Bridge (see page 166).
- Thoracic Twist (see page 79) or Child's Twist (see page 147).

Pranayama and *Savasana*

- Counting the Breaths (see page 243) or Ratio Breathing (see page 253).
- Choose a *Savasana* option (see page 206).

A Practice for Freedom and Connection

In this sequence we move from side to side to fire up the cross-connections and side connections in the body. You might find that you come off your mat and face different directions.

Opening

- Start lying down. Breath Attention (see page 241) (1–2 minutes).
- Wake up the face and jaw by moving the tongue, jaw and brow, then turn the head from side to side.

Preparation

- Passive Knees-to-Chest Pose (see page 199).
- Active Knees-to-Chest Pose (see page 199), taking the knees from side to side.
- Supine Twist to right (see page 201), open up the left arm.
- Lift left knee and Supine Twist to the left, open up right arm.
- Repeat from side to side 2–3 times.
- From the right-hand side, push to sit, Lounging Pigeon with right knee forward (see page 189), gentle hip circles.
- Tuck knees in, lie down, roll from side to side again.
- Repeat rolling to the left with left knee forward in Lounging Pigeon.

Transition and Warm-Up

- Lounging Pigeon to Windscreen Wipers (see page 224).
- Plant left hand, swing right leg round to Side Plank A (see page 134), making arm circles, then bring hands under shoulders.
- All Fours Curtsey (see page 140).
- Advanced Cow/Cat (see page 220) – option for Child's Pose (see page 145).
- Superman (see page 143) – hip circles, knee to opposite elbow (right leg).
- Twisted Lunge (see page 105) – step right foot forward, explore circles with the top arm, maybe lift the back knee.
- Bring right foot further back and find the outside edge of the back foot for Side Plank B (see page 135), lifting up and down x 3.
- Sit down and unwind the legs to lie down and repeat on the other side.

Dynamic Standing Poses

- Down Dog (see page 148) and roll up to stand.
- Standing Pigeon with right leg lifted (see page 113).
- Step the right leg back and allow the hips to follow for High Lunge (see page 107).
- Push off the front foot and open out to Horse Pose (see page 123): option for Eagle Arms (see page 124).
- Turn to the back of the mat and find Twisted Lunge, with the right knee bent, left hand to the floor.
- Step back to Down Dog, Advanced Cow/Cat or Rolling *Vinyasa* (see page 222).
- Repeat 2–3 times with right leg lifted.
- On final round, from Twisted Lunge, move to Side Plank B or Full Side Plank (see page 136).
- Repeat on the other side.

Closing

- Reclined *Baddha Konasana* (see page 209).
- Supported Bridge (see page 169) or Supported Fish (see page 197).

Pranayama and *Savasana*

- Alternate Nostril Breathing (see page 254).
- Choose a *Savasana* (see page 206) option.

A Practice to Explore Spirals

We are made up of spirals and there are no straight lines in our bodies. This practice is about allowing the movement and poses to make us aware of how the body is one integrated piece.

Opening

- Start lying down. Breath Attention or Simple Passive Breathing (see page 241) (1–2 minutes).
- Wake up the face and jaw by moving the tongue, jaw and brow, then turn the head from side to side.

Preparation

- Windscreen Wipers (see page 224).
- Rest on the back, then Knees-to-Chest Pose (see page 199) and rock from side to side.
- Sitting in Easy Pose (see page 170), Eagle Arms with right over left (see page 180). Circle in both directions, then come to pause somewhere that feels useful to you and take 3–4 breaths.
- Repeat with left arm over right.
- Lean back and shake out the legs, if needed.

Transition and Warm-Up

- Low Lunge with right foot forward (see page 104).
- Line up the front heel with the back knee and swing the back ankle in, so the torso is open to the side.
- Place right elbow on right knee and side reach with left arm, then spiral. Repeat 2–3 times. Pause.
- Bring the left arm to the floor, sweep it around to find Side Plank A (see page 134).
- Bend the outstretched leg so that you can push up to Low Lunge and then repeat.
- After 2–3 rounds, pause in Side Plank A, walking the hands underneath the shoulders.
- All Fours Curtsey with the right leg going behind (see page 140), pushing into the foot to pulse gently; pause and breathe.
- Advanced Cow/Cat (see page 220).
- Repeat with the left leg in front.

Dynamic Standing Poses

- Chair Pose (see page 128) to Angry Animal with the right leg lifted (see page 113).
- Step the right leg back, and allow the hips to follow for High Lunge (see page 107). Bend and Lengthen the legs a few times (see page 110).
- Push off the front foot and open to Horse Pose (see page 123).
- Add Eagle Arms (see page 124) – start small and pause, then come up to centre, release the elbows.
- Step the left foot behind the right into Standing Curtsey (see page 126).
- Move from Horse Pose to Standing Curtsey a few times, before pausing in the curtsey.
- Bring the left elbow over the right for Eagle Arms and breathe here.
- Can you unspiral yourself? Practise winding up and unwinding a couple of times.
- Forward Fold (see page 98) to a *Vinyasa* option (see page 220), then Down Dog, Forward Fold, and roll up to stand.
- Repeat on the other side.

Closing

- Basic Bridge (see page 166).
- Choice of twist on the back.

Pranayama and *Savasana*

- Nine-Part Breath (see page 244), using awareness of the spirals to find space for the breath.
- Choose a *Savasana* (see page 206) option.

A Practice to Counteract Sitting All Day

Most of us sit for long periods, which can lead to a compressed front body,
an overstretched back body and compromised breathing. In this sequence we
actively work to engage the back body to help open the front.

Opening

- Belly Lying *Savasana* (see page 208). Allow the belly to relax, notice how it is to be on your front. Allow the jaw, head and throat to relax, and the armpits to open, the hips and thighs to soften (2–3 minutes).

Preparation

- All Fours Hip Circles (see page 139), gentle Cow/Cat (see page 144).
- Engage Ocean Breath (see page 242) as you move.
- All Fours Rib Circles (see page 139): imagine you are in a barrel and are trying to clean the inside using only your ribs.
- Kneeling Cow-Faced Shoulder Opener (see page 182), turning the head gently and then pausing. Repeat on both sides.
- Child's Pose (see page 145) – notice how it feels to be in this pose.

Transition and Warm-Up

- Rolling up to high kneeling from Child's Pose, engage the legs and torso to lift and control the movement. Repeat 3–4 times.
- Elastic Lunge (see page 106). Repeat 3–4 times.
- Lazy Tail Wag (see page 95).
- All Fours Chest Opener (see page 140) for 2–3 breaths.
- Advanced Cow/Cat (see page 220) x 1–2 rounds.
- Wide-arm Swimming Cobra (see page 154).
- Start to walk the arms in to Sphinx (see page 157), then turn the head and relax the jaw.
- Forearm Plank (see page 133), push the heels back and the hands down, hip circles.
- Child's Pose to rest, then repeat on the other side.

Dynamic Standing Poses

- Advanced Cow/Cat or Rolling *Vinyasa* (see page 222).
- Down Dog (see page 148), then Three-Legged Dog (see page 150), pulsing off the back leg to step the lifted leg forward.
- High Lunge with right leg back (see page 107).
- Reverse Warrior (see page 102), bring hands behind the head, lift the head, relax the arms.
- Horse Pose (see page 123), then find Cactus Arms (see page 179), engaging the mid-back.
- Surfer (see page 127) and twist the torso toward the bent knee, keeping the elbows still, then move to the other side. Repeat 2–3 times on each side.
- Turn to High Lunge with right leg forward.
- Down Dog to Rolling *Vinyasa* or Advanced Cow/Cat.
- Option for Rockstar (see page 164).
- Lie down or Child's Pose to pause.
- Repeat on the other side.

Closing

- Supported Bridge with hands on the lower ribs (see page 169) and breathe here.
- Supine Twist (see page 200) .
- Bound Angle Pose (see page 204) or Reclined *Baddha Konasana* (see page 209).

Pranayama and *Savasana*

- Three-Part Breath (see page 242) lying down, activating parts of the lungs and opening the chest.
- Choose a *Savasana* option (see page 206).

A Gentle Practice to Connect to the Emotional Body

This practice encourages us to connect with each of our emotional *chakras* (see page 248). Some places will feel more open, or easier to connect to, and you might feel emotional in some poses. If things get too uncomfortable, come out of the pose, take a few moments and go back if you feel okay to do so.

Muladhara

- The base *chakra* is your connection to earth and grounding energy. It is located at the pelvic floor. In each pose, bring your attention to the legs and feet, and imagine drawing up earth energy into the pelvic floor.
- Forward Fold (see page 98).
- Squat (see page 130).
- Forward Fold.

Svadhisthana

- The sacral *chakra* is located just below the belly button, but further back in the pelvis. This is the seat of your desire. Breathe down into the pelvic area in each pose; you can also visualize a ball of light at the centre of the pelvis.
- Lounging Pigeon (see page 189) or Half Pigeon (see page 190).
- Low Lunge (see page 104).
- Twisted Lunge (see page 105).

Manipura

- Located at the solar plexus, the solar plexus *chakra* is the centre of digestion and fire. In the pose, visualize a ball of yellow fire at the solar plexus and, when you breathe into it, imagine it glowing and burning brightly.
- Thoracic Twist lying down (see page 79).

Anahata

- The heart *chakra*, located at the base of the heart, in the centre of the chest, is your emotional centre. In the poses you can breathe down into the base of the heart.
- All Fours Chest Opener (see page 140).
- Sphinx (see page 157).

Vishuddha

- The energy centre at the throat is related to your need for expression. Take care that the back of the neck feels okay in this pose, and support the head, if needed. Breathe into the throat and neck, imagining that you are a fish with gills.
- Supported Fish (see page 197).

Ajna

- This is the seat of your intuition, located behind the eyes in the mid-brain. Soften the eyes and brow, and allow your attention to rest in the space behind the eyes.
- Child's Pose with bolster (see page 145).
- Supported Bridge (see page 168).

Sahaswara

- Located at the crown of the head, the crown *chakra* is your connection to the divine.
- Legs Up the Wall (see page 194) or Supported Shoulder Stand (see page 193).
- Choose a *Savasana* option (see page 206).

A Gentle Flow for Boundaries

Boundaries are essential for us in order to navigate life. In this sequence the props are used to create a boundary so that we can really soften and surrender. Notice how putting the boundary in place releases the stress in the body.

Props: a bolster or 2–3 large firm cushions or pillows, some blocks, a blanket, a strap, warm comfy clothes and a timer.

Opening

- Lie on your back and bring attention to your body.
- Allow the floor to be a natural boundary to the back of the body and give your weight to it.
- Notice how it feels to be supported by the floor. Stay for 5 minutes.

Reclined *Baddha Konasana*

- Reclined *Baddha Konasana* (see page 209): bring cushions or blocks under the knees so the legs are supported. Stay in the pose for 3–5 minutes.
- Counterpose: gentle Forward Fold (see page 98) or Windscreen Wipers (see page 224).

Child's Twist

- Child's Twist (see page 147). Notice how the bolster under the body allows for a full sense of opening and softening.
- Counterpose: Cow/Cat (see page 144) or All Fours Hip Circles (see page 139).

Forward Fold

- Forward Fold. Put a bolster or fat cushion under your knees so that the legs can let go. Bring another bolster under your head, so that you relax the head and neck. If you don't have a large enough bolster or cushion, you can use a chair or coffee table.
- Counterpose: Windscreen Wipers, leaning back on the hands to lift and open the chest.

Sphinx

- Sphinx (see page 157): put a bolster or cushion under the armpits so that the upper body can relax. Stay for another 1–2 minutes only.
- Counterpose: a gentle Child's Pose, moving the hips and snaking the spine softly.

All Fours Chest Opener

- All Fours Chest Opener (see page 140) over a bolster: put a bolster or large cushion under your chest so that you can give your weight to it.
- Counterpose: gentle Child's Pose, bringing the arms alongside the lower legs.

Reclining Hand to Big Toe

- Find Your 60 Per Cent (see page 47).
- Counterpose: Knees-to-Chest Pose (see page 198).

Lying Side Bend

- Lying Side Bend (see page 198).
- Counterpose: Knees-to-Chest Pose, full-body stretch, Windscreen Wipers or anything else gentle that the body needs, before settling down again on the mat.

Savasana

- Choose a *Savasana* option (see page 206).

The Three *Gunas*

One of the most enjoyable things about developments in yoga is where ancient philosophy meets modern science. One area where they align is the system of the Three Gunas. Originating from Samkhya philosophy, the *gunas* describe three states of reality (*tattvas*). Everything in the material world – from humans right through to natural phenomena, food and matter – is said to have one of these qualities. *Sattva* is light, balanced and white in colour; *Rajas* is fiery and energetic and red; and *Tamas* is inert, heavy and black.

We can start to apply these qualities more specifically to how the body is regulated through the nervous system and how this appears in our state of mind, and in how our muscles and joints are expressed. *Rajas* is when we are stimulated and move into our stress response. *Tamas* is when we are shut down and switching off. *Sattva* is when we are alert but relaxed and in balance.

In both a *Tamasic* and *Sattvic* state we are in our Parasympathetic Nervous System, but different parts of it: *Tamas* is the "play dead" side of our early threat response, while *Sattva* is the social, connected, soothing side; it is also a response to stress, but a more balanced one, where we seek friends and family to support and help us, and where we attend a yoga class to connect with others and ourselves. *Rajas* is where our Sympathetic Nervous System, or fight-and-flight mode, is activated.

How we feel, via fascia and the nervous system, has a direct effect on our physical bodies. When we are *Rajasic* or in fight-and-flight mode, we might be tense and rigid, especially if our joints are locked out. When we are *Tamasic* the body is collapsed, with no muscle tension or engagement. In a *Sattvic* state there is muscle engagement and tone where needed, but also a sense of relaxation. The body is buoyant, pliable and fluid.

Rajasic

1. Standing up, lock out one leg and make it rigid. Then try to walk around the room.

2. Notice what patterns occur throughout the body as you walk with this locked-out leg.

3. You might notice tension creeping up into the hips and back as your gait is affected.

4. You can repeat this with locked-out arms or a clenched jaw.

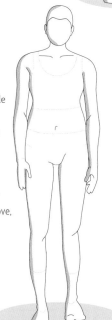

Tamasic

1. Now collapse as much as you can while standing: slouch the shoulders, round the back and then try to walk again.

2. Notice the impact on your ability to move, as well as on your energy levels.

Sattvic

1. Now see if you can find a balance between these, where the muscles are engaged but not rigid.

2. The knees might be softly bent, the feet engaged, with a sense of coiled springiness in the body.

3. You can shift your weight comfortably from foot to foot and with balance.

4. There is some tension, but you can move with ease.

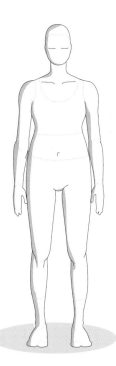

Moving Between States

The yoga therapist Ann Swanson uses a dial diagram that conveys how we move between these states, depending on the environment; how well we self-regulate and use support to assist us. She says to think of it like a dimmer-switch for lighting – able to move back and forth. Ideally we are looking to spend more time in a *Sattvic* state: resting, connecting, with some excitement, fun and exercise as we move more into a gentle *Rajasic* state. When we rest and sleep we come into a *Tamasic* state: the body is heavy and unmoveable.

If we go too far into a *Rajasic* state we might experience anger or anxiety; too much into a *Tamasic* state and we may begin to feel hopeless or withdrawn. This shows how there is a strong link between an anxious and depressed state, moving from *Rajasic* to *Tamasic* on the right-hand side of the dial. While we know that sleep and rest are vital for us, when triggered from a *Tamasic* state and not a *Sattvic* one, we see that problems of lethargy and withdrawal can arise.

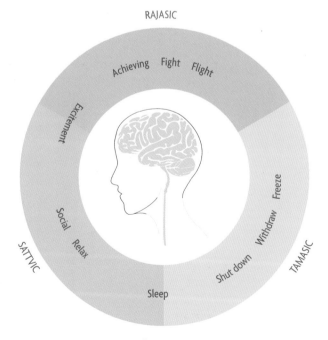

Sympathetic nervous system

RAJASIC

Achieving   Fight   Flight

Excitement

Freeze

Withdraw

Shut down

Social

Relax

SATTVIC

TAMASIC

Sleep

Parasympathetic nervous system

Using *Pranayama* and Visualization in Practice

In this section we will employ some simple *pranayama* techniques, sometimes alongside other subtle-body practices, to illustrate how they can be used in a practical way. They build on the idea of the *vayus* or Five Winds (see page 252) as we move *prana* or energy around the body. Allow 5–10 minutes for each practice.

All of these practices are done seated, with a long spine and a soft face, eyes and jaw. You can sit back against the wall or on a chair, but avoid slumping. Start with 1–2 minutes of soft Ocean Breath (see page 242), perhaps with a small pause between the inhale and exhale, and vice versa.

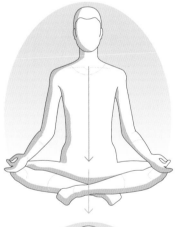

Grounding (Related *Vayu: Apana*)

Use when you need grounding, connection to the earth and support.

- **Inhale**: draw the breath down to the pelvic floor.
- **Exhale**: as you breathe out, visualize the breath going down into the earth beneath you.

Option: imagine a light moving down with the inhale and out into the earth as you breathe out.

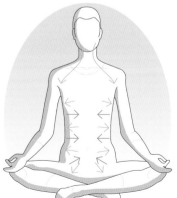

Restoring (Related *Vayu: Prana*)

Use when you need quiet and introspection, are feeling overwhelmed or over-stimulated.

- **Inhale**: feel the whole torso gently expand – the chest, ribs, belly; back, side and front.
- **Exhale**: allow the air to leave physically, but visualize the energy or *prana* staying inside.

Option: you can also visualize light filling the body on the inhale, and staying in the whole body even as you exhale.

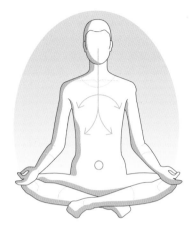

Digesting (Related *Vayu: Samana*)

Use when you need to process or digest emotions, feelings, thoughts and events.

- **Inhale**: breathe into the belly, the sides and back as well as the belly front.
- **Exhale**: visualize the energy or *prana* moving into a ball of bright light in the solar plexus.
- **Inhale**: breathe into the belly, the sides and back as well as the belly front.
- **Exhale**: visualize the ball of bright light spreading out through the body, burning up all that is no longer needed.

Option: as you exhale, gently draw the belly button in for *Uddiyana Bandha* (see page 258).

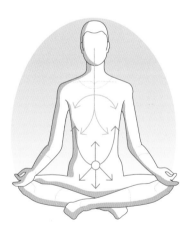

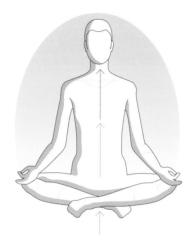

Uplifting (Related *Vayu: Udana*)

Use when you need energizing, feel sluggish or in a low mood.

- **Inhale**: draw the breath up from the earth into the pelvic floor.
- **Exhale**: send the breath and *prana* up through the crown of the head.

Options: on the inhale, gently lift the pelvic floor into the *Mula Bandha* (see page 259) for a pause, then release as you exhale upward. You can also visualize drawing light up from the earth into the body through the pelvic floor, and exhaling the light up through the crown of the head.

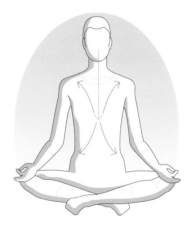

Centring (Related *Vayu: Vyana*)

Use when you need to centre and come back to the heart and body or connect with yourself again.

- **Inhale**: bring the breath down to the base of the heart, the mid-chest.
- **Exhale**: send the *prana* out into the whole body.

Option: again you can visualize a light accompanying the breath.

Practices for Relaxation

If you recall the concept of the *gunas* – the nervous-system dial (see page 278) – you'll see that it's easy to go from being really stressed to collapsing. Many of us mistake the "sofa slump" for true relaxation, and it's easy to use maladaptive coping strategies such as alcohol or shopping to manage stress. However, watching TV or any other screen is not relaxing for the nervous system, as we are still being stimulated, even while slumped on the sofa.

True relaxation can be hard for many of us. If we are in that "wired" state for long periods, to come into a relaxed state with no distractions may sometimes feel frightening. Even if we are able to relax the body, we might find that the mind is still buzzing like a radio and we can't switch off. And even if we can find a moment of quiet, it can be disconcerting, because that is when we start to hear all the things that are kept hidden by our constant busyness.

But real relaxation is critical to enable our nervous system to recalibrate, our brain to process information and our body to recuperate. This rest is not sleep, although these practices can be done before bed to aid sleep, if needed. But you can do them any time: just make sure they are done with the intention to relax and rest. Set up your space with soft lighting and music, and maybe a candle. Wear comfortable clothes that you can move and breathe freely in; if practising in the evening after a long day at work, a shower to wash away the day can also help.

This isn't a sequence – rather some suggestions for practices that you can do to relax. You'll need a mat, cushions or a bolster and a blanket.

Poses

If you feel agitated or anxious, it can help to move for 10–15 minutes to shift adrenaline from the body. This might involve an Advanced Cow/Cat (see page 220) or some Rolling *Vinyasas* (see page 222), rolling from side to side into a twist, or some Low Lunges (see page 104) into Down Dog (see page 148). Finish in a lying position.

You may want to take some passive poses as well as, or instead of, these. They can all be done lying down, such as a twist or Lying Side Bend (see page 198). If you have been sitting all day, perhaps a Supported Bridge (see page 169) or a Sphinx (see page 157) to open the front body is a good idea.

Restorative poses are the best for relaxation: try Reclined *Baddha Konasana* (see page 209), Legs Up the Wall (see page 194) or a twist over a bolster.

Breathing

Use these exercises either on their own or in a restorative pose. You can do them sitting or lying down: deep Tummy Breathing (see page 238), Three-Part Breath (see page 242), lengthening the exhale.

Meditation

Yoga Nidra is one of the best meditation practices for deep relaxation: but you do need a recording, so I would suggest finding one online or using a meditation app. Then you can play it and simply listen: remember to stay awake as best you can!

Savasana

Even if your whole practice has been about relaxing, you must always leave time for a 5–10-minute *Savasana* so that your nervous system and body can process it and you can experience deep rest. It takes time to come into a relaxed state, and it might not be until *Savasana* that you can finally be still.

Things You Can Do in Bed

Some poses work well in bed, such as Knees-to-Chest Pose (see page 199), twists done on the floor and Bound Angle Bridge (see page 168). You can sit on your pillows for a Seated Forward Fold (see page 175) or Seated Twist (see page 173). You can also do Legs Up the Wall (see page 194) with your hips on the pillows and your legs on the headboard or wall. Often I will practise lengthening my exhales in bed, just before I fall asleep.

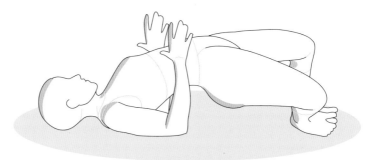

Bound Angle Bridge

Practices for Stress Management

Managing stress is a big driver for people taking up yoga, and research shows that the various yoga practices can be beneficial. It's important to remember that some stress is needed in life for a sense of vitality and excitement, and that we stress our systems in many different ways during the day. It's when we can't turn the dial back down again, and find time to really switch off and relax, that stress can become a chronic problem.

In yoga philosophy, much of our stress is said to be mind-created – it's how we perceive and respond to stress, which may depend on the stories, beliefs and patterns that have been generated in us over time. Understanding how your thoughts about a stressful event can affect its impact on you can help, and strategies such as Cognitive Behavioural Therapy use a similar approach to this. When we can experience what an alternative possibility feels like in the body, we allow ourselves to be more open to it actually happening.

Meditation practices can help with sitting with your thoughts and feelings and noticing them as they arise. Such a practice can provide space around your inner landscape so that you can see what's actually true for you, as well as what helps. Meditation doesn't have to involve 15–20 minutes of sitting. Just take a moment to feel the breath on the upper lip, or in the belly, and ask, "What is going on for me right now?", then acknowledge your thoughts and feelings. With persistent unhelpful thinking, you can ask, "Is that really true? How does believing that thought makes me feel? How it would it be if I let it go?" These questions, devised by the American speaker and author Byron Katie, lie at the heart of her work Loving What Is, and the same approach also forms the basis of therapies such as Acceptance and Commitment Therapy.

We also need to feel and process our emotions. When we have unpleasant or difficult emotions, our instinctive response is to push them away, keep them locked down inside us or pretend they're not there. For many of us, this is a learned response from childhood, where we understood from our parents that certain emotions were not allowed. When we don't acknowledge and digest what we really feel, that stress gets stuck in the body in a low-level form, impacting on the nervous system, our tissues and the subtle-energy body. We have to acknowledge all the different facets of our lives and understand what they mean for us, in order to manage stress well.

As stress has such a physical effect on the body, moving and breathing can be direct ways to lessen the impact. Moving is especially important if the body is full of adrenaline: however, many people add to their stress load by choosing hard-hitting or extreme exercise regimes. We need to include more gentle movement in our schedules to allow the nervous system to dial down. As we have seen in the Breath section (pages 232–245), there is a direct relationship between the breath and our nervous system, so we can utilize a range of breathing techniques to dial back the stress response.

If we look back at the *gunas* and our stress dial (see page 278), we see the importance of the social vagus nerve in managing stress. This means that other activities that involve socializing and connecting to others are important for us. It might mean coffee with a friend, joining an online support forum or in-person group, or finding a meditation class or movement session. Being with others, sharing an experience and connecting in some way, is a powerful stress reliever.

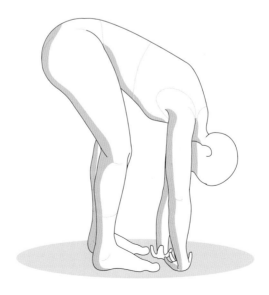

Forward Fold

Daily Movement

Daily life for many is sedentary and repetitive. To counteract this we need to move our bodies in different ways throughout the day. The key is to take time to step back from our tasks and thought processes to assess how our bodies feel and what kind of movement is needed.

When you wake up, start by wiggling, squirming and stretching to allow your body to come online. Supine Twist (see page 201), Knees-to-Chest Pose (see page 199) or Windscreen Wipers (see page 224) will all wake your system gently.

Before, during or after showering you can do Forward Fold (see page 98), Chair Pose (see page 128) or Hunchback (see page 129) and come up and down on your tip toes. Some High Lunges (see pages 107–110) and Warriors (see pages 100–103 and 114) will also help generate energy and vitality in the body and make you feel ready for the day.

If you have a desk-based job, make sure your computer, desk and chair are set up correctly so that you can work comfortably. Periodically, lift your gaze, do a Seated Twist (see page 173), Seated Cow/Cat (see page 172) and Seated Pigeon (see page 190). Stretch your arms over your head, turn your head and roll your shoulders. Also, remember to stand up and walk around, even if it's just to go to the kitchen or bathroom.

Physical work makes a lot of demands on the body: sawing, chopping, lifting, bending and reaching are all done repetitively with awareness on the task rather than the feeling in the body. Take time to make opposite movements to the ones you do a lot and make sure to use the other side of your body too. Parenting young children can also be physically demanding, with lots of bending, lifting and carrying. Make sure to check in with your body and balance out movements.

Break time or the middle of the day are good times to do some more deliberate movements. Many yoga poses can be done using a chair or table, such as Down Dog (see page 148), Updog (see page 158) or lunging with a foot on a chair. A break is also a great time to go outside for a walk: choose a lunch place further away from your place of work, and take the stairs.

Before you go to bed, try restorative poses on your back (see pages 169 and 192–197) and slower movements to help your body wind down for sleep. You can even do some poses on your bed, such as Legs Up the Wall (see page 194).

Daily Breathing

We can work with our breathing to bring about different states, and this works well as we move throughout our day. Certain practices will be more stimulating or uplifting, while others are more calming.

Waking Up: Tibetan Cleansing

In the morning we want to wake up and get the system going, but not kick ourselves into overdrive. This technique calms the mind, brings attention to the breath and balances us, ready for the day ahead. Adding the arm movements to the breath means there is a lot to concentrate on, so there is less space for the mind to wander.

1. Start by tuning into the breath, then allow it to settle into its own rhythm: not forcing or pushing.
2. Notice the inhale/pause/exhale/pause pattern to the breath – follow this for several rounds.
3. Find Chin or *Jnana Mudra* (see page 256) by bringing the tip of the index fingers to the tips of the thumbs.
4. Inhale: lift the right hand up.
5. Pause: bring the right middle finger to the right nostril and close it off.
6. Exhale: keep the finger on the right nostril and exhale through the left, while lowering the elbow.
7. Pause: lower the right hand to the thigh.
8. Repeat on the other side.
9. Repeat for 3–5 minutes (set a timer) or 30 rounds.

Other options: Alternate Nostril Breathing (see page 254), Ocean Breath (see page 242), Ratio Breathing (see page 253), Shining Skull Breath (see page 253).

During a Meeting/When Needing to Focus

Focus and attention are interesting because they can often tip the balance so that we end up in our stress response. These attitudes are on the cusp of the dial between the social Sattvic state and the Rajasic stress response (see page 278), so care is needed that we don't go too far into fight-or-flight mode.

Breath awareness involves paying attention to your breath on the upper lip, in the nostrils or in the belly. Notice its length, texture and rhythm. If you get distracted, don't worry: just start again on the next breath. See if you can keep part of your attention on the breath, as well as listening to the conversation in a meeting or whatever else you need to focus on.

Other options: Counting the Breaths (see page 243): inhale one, exhale one, and so on; rectangular breathing, Ocean Breath (see page 242).

Impending Deadline/Too Many To-Dos/Feeling Frazzled

When we feel that dial turn too much toward our stress response, we need help dialling it back down again. Deliberately lengthening the exhale will help. Start by counting your natural breath and seeing the average length of the inhale; then make your exhale one count longer. Keep repeating this for a couple of minutes. You can also play with it by making the exhale two or three counts longer: remember to keep the practice soft and without pushing. Pushing only makes us more stressed!

After Lunch/Needing to Energize

When we're relaxed, our breathing is much more passive. To energize, we can stimulate the nervous system by making the breath more active. Ocean Breath (see page 242) is great for this. If you have had a big lunch, you might need to wait half an hour or longer before you change your breathing: this allows the body to start the digestion process and for you to feel much less full. Do not contract the belly on the exhale with a tummy full of food!

Other options: Shining Skull Breath (see page 253) is very stimulating, but needs to be done on an empty stomach! Getting up for a walk, or moving and stretching, will also help.

In Bed

At night-time we want to soothe and calm our system, ready for sleep.

Polarity breathing is a simple breathing and visualization technique to do lying down. Simply inhale and visualize the breath going down to your feet; exhale, visualizing the breath going up to the head. Repeat for several minutes or until you drop off.

Other options: deep Tummy Breathing (see page 238), Counting the Breaths (see page 243) and Extending the Exhale (see page 243) are all calming before sleep.

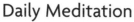

Daily Meditation

Meditation takes time and practice, but it doesn't have to take a long time! All of these practices can be done in ten minutes. Set your timer: if you have an intermittent chime sound, this is good for bringing you back if the mind wanders – which it will do!

Preparation for All Meditations

1. Sit upright, lower back supported, feet planted, and allow your tongue, jaw and eyes to soften; if the eyes are open, allow the gaze to soften too.
2. Draw your attention to your breathing. There is no need to force or push the breath. Let it finds its natural rhythm for a few rounds, and then start to lengthen it slightly, maybe by 2 or 3 per cent.
3. Breathe into your belly, lower back and chest and exhale.

Centring

This is for coming back to yourself – to the core of your being. It is good after a stressful day, or first thing in the morning to prepare for the day ahead.

1. With your eyes closed or half open, visualize, imagine or sense a central channel through your body: from the crown of the head in front of the spine, down to the pelvic floor. The channel goes down through your seat, the floor and into the earth; it also goes up through the top of your head out into the world. Sit for a moment with this image or feeling.
2. As you inhale, visualize, imagine or sense golden light coming up from the earth into your central channel. You can engage the pelvic floor (using the *Mula Bandha*, see page 259) to contain the energy.
3. As you exhale, this golden light goes up the channel, through the crown of the head into the world. Keep repeating, in your own time. If the mind wanders you can add a mantra, such as "So" on the inhale and "Hum" on the exhale, to help you focus.
4. When your alarm goes off, release the visualization and rest where you are. Keep the breath soft and notice how you feel. Remain sitting with awareness for as long as you need.

Body Scan

This mindfulness meditation is great for when you are disconnected from yourself and need to check in with how you feel.

1. Take your attention to each part of the body and let it rest there, noticing what there is to feel – even if you don't feel anything, or it is numb or tingling, or there is pressure or touch; then move on to the next area.
2. Start with the feet, ankles and lower legs; the thighs, hips and buttocks; belly and lower back, chest and upper back; arms and hands, neck and shoulders; head and face. This is where a timer with an intermittent ping helps, as you can set it for one-minute intervals and move on to the next part of the body when it sounds.
3. Finish with awareness of the whole body and some Ocean Breathing (see page 242) to ground yourself.

Watching Thoughts

We can't make the monkey-mind be quiet, but we can change our relationship to it. In this mindfulness meditation you practise looking at your thoughts, rather than being in them.

1. Start with some simple breath awareness and feeling the breath in the body. You can start with Counting the Breaths (see page 243), Ocean Breath (see page 242) or Three-Part Breath (see page 242).
2. Once breathing is established and you feel centred, allow your mind to become a TV screen, and thoughts to be images and videos being played on the screen. You are the watcher of the screen, not actively involved in the images. Stay for 3–5 minutes, allowing each thought to pass on the screen of your mind. Some might linger, others will be fleeting. Notice if you get drawn into the narrative: can you stay in the audience, watching?
3. If you get drawn in, you can come back to the feeling of the breath in the body, or the sense of sitting on the chair or cushion, and start again.
4. Notice how you feel about the thoughts as you remove yourself from the storyline: do you feel differently?

Grounding

This brings attention and energy down into the pelvis and base of the spine, helping you feel grounded, secure and supported – good when you feel overwhelmed or over-stimulated.

1. Bring your attention to the tip of your nose. Notice the breath in the nostrils. Watch how the breath comes in your nostrils, and visualize or sense it going to the top of your head. As you breathe out, watch the breath travel down the spine into the lower back. Return to the tip of the nose: inhaling, the breath goes to the top of the head; exhaling, the breath goes down the spine to the lower back. Keep repeating.
2. Keep the breath and eyes soft and, as best you can, try not to move your eyes up and down. Visualize, sense or imagine the breath travelling up to the top of the head and down into the lower back. Don't rush your breath. Notice any tendencies to force or push; allow the flow of breath to be easy, as far as possible.
3. As you exhale, allow the sensation of breath to collect in the lower body, offering a rooting and grounding sensation.
4. Repeat as many times as feels comfortable, then stop the visualization and just sit, with your attention resting behind your eyes, with soft breathing.
5. Come out of the meditation when you are ready.

Heart-Centred

This is good if you are feeling low, lonely, disconnected and separate.

1. Bring the hands into Lotus or *Padma Mudra* or Fearless Heart Mudra (see page 257) against the chest.
2. Connect to your breathing for 1–2 minutes, allowing it to get a little slower and deeper.
3. Bring your attention into the base of the heart/middle of the chest/sternum.
4. Visualize or sense the breath coming in through the nose and down into the base of the heart as you inhale. As you exhale, it goes back up and out through the nose. Repeat for 1–2 minutes.
5. Inhale down to the heart; you might visualize a bright white lotus flower opening up in the heart space. Exhale, and the lotus closes a little and the breath goes back up and out. You can even make the movements with your hands, opening and closing the palms a little. Repeat for 2–3 minutes.
6. Now allow the breath to relax completely and bring your attention to the heart centre. Allow it to stay there and notice what you experience for 1–2 minutes.

Dealing with Difficult Emotions

Our default approach to difficult emotions is either to bury them or push them away. This is a survival strategy born of our hard-wiring, which senses that anything unpleasant is a threat. As we live longer, more complex lives, we need ways of processing and digesting what we feel. If we don't do this, emotions, experiences and events get stuck in our nervous systems and tissues.

In yoga we practise turning toward our difficulties and allowing them to be there. We acknowledge that things might be hard for us at the moment, that we feel sad or angry, disappointed or resentful. We then practise softening toward our experience and allowing ourselves to fully accept it and process it. This might be uncomfortable, but it is so important to allow real connection to ourselves and to move through things. This idea of emotional digestion is adapted from classical Tantric yoga via the scholar-practitioner Christopher Wallis.

Notice where you feel the emotion in the body: is there a heaviness, ache or blockage somewhere? Does a particular place feel numb? Choose a restorative pose. Some ideas might include: Child's Pose (see page 145) for grounding and calming; chest openers for expression and heart connection; twists for emotions felt in the gut; inversions for intuition and insight.

Progressively relax your body: start with your feet and work up your body to the face. Wherever you feel tension or gripping, either adjust your position or wriggle, fidget and soften until the body can surrender completely. Then relax the face: the jaw and tongue; swallow to relax the throat; soften the eye sockets, eyeballs and brow. Allow your mind to soften: you can't stop thinking, but you can turn the noise down a little. Then bring your attention back to the body and notice what arises emotionally. It might appear as a physical sensation. Can you allow it to be there? If you can, softly and kindly breathe into what you feel by softening your approach to whatever you experience, it becomes possible to have it there inside you. As you notice your emotions and breathe gently into them, you may find they become less difficult; or perhaps you need to cry or they might become stronger. If at any time the process becomes too uncomfortable, come back to your breath.

You can come out of the pose whenever you're ready: it isn't a failure to want to stop the exercise; in fact it is an act of awareness and self-care. You can always start again another time, if it feels right to do so. You might need to lie or sit comfortably for five minutes at the end to reground and settle.

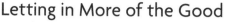

Letting in More of the Good

Apart from big events such as birthdays, weddings and holidays, most of the good things we experience are small: the sunlight on your face after several grey days; the warm cup of coffee on your break; the beautiful autumn or spring colours; a child's laughter; your favourite tune coming on the car radio; a hug from a friend; that moment when you lie down on your yoga mat.

These small, pleasurable moments are really easy to miss. Yoga helps us develop our awareness so that we can be more mindful of them as they arise. It is in delving into the nuances of each moment that we can experience real joy: take time to drink the coffee, savour its smell, flavour and warmth; don't distract yourself with your phone or other device; take refuge in the moment of quiet that your break brings you; sit outside with your coffee, if possible, bringing in other sensations, such as light and nature. This pleasurable experience might only last five minutes, but it will be one worth savouring.

When practising yoga, make a ritual out of it. I always shower before practising, to wash away the day or the night before, and put on clean practice clothes. Light a candle or put on some music. Even if you're using a video or app, try not to let yourself be distracted by the phone or device: turn off other notifications, so that you can fully immerse yourself. In a group class, switch off your phone before entering the room, and arrive a little early so that you have time to settle on the mat. Chatting to friends at classes also boosts the social vagus and helps alleviate stress, so enjoy those moments too.

Gratitude is another element in immersing ourselves in the good. When we take time to acknowledge what we are thankful for – no matter how small – we extend the pleasure of those moments, and they get remembered in our systems. Not only does this counteract stress, but it makes it more likely that we'll seek out these experiences again. If you know how good a particular class makes you feel, and deeply acknowledge your gratitude at being able to attend, there is more chance you'll create another opportunity to attend.

At the end of each evening, you can write down three things you are grateful for that day, focusing on how they made you feel and what you noticed about them: colours, smells, texture, taste. An example might be: "I am so very grateful to watch TV for 20 minutes with the kids: hearing their laughter, watching their smiles, feeling their bodies against mine and experiencing our love for one another."

Glossary

Abhinivesha: clinging to life

Abhyasa: practice

Ahimsa: non-violence

Ananda: bliss

Aparigraha: non-greed

Asana: traditionally, a seated posture for meditation; today, a pose, movement and shape for physical yoga

Ascetic: a man who has renounced everyday life and its comforts to live outside the community and dedicate himself to his practice of yoga

Ashtanga: the Eight-Limbed Path of yoga; also a form of athletic postural yoga

Asmita: the wrong perception of self

Atman: the inner, individual self or soul

Avidya: ignorance, wrong knowledge

Bhakti yoga: the yoga of devotion, a religious path

Brahman: the ultimate unchanging reality; the universal self

Brahmanism: religious practices and thought pertaining to the priestly class in India; also denotes the parts of Hinduism that stayed close to these teachings, especially those directly descended from the Vedic period

Citta: heart–mind

Darshana: worldview, philosophy

Deity: a god or goddess considered divine

Dharma: right action and purpose, in terms of both duty and life after death

Dhyana: absorption with continuity

Diksha: initiation (into a Tantric lineage)

Dualism: a worldview that there are two or more fundamentally distinct and irreconcilable essences to reality, e.g. consciousness vs matter

Dvesha: aversion

Hatha yoga: the period of yoga in late medieval times focused on the movement of energy in the body to acquire special powers and achieve liberation; can also refer to a slower form of modern postural yoga

Householder: non-ascetic, regular community-dwelling person, with a family and job

Jainism: an early Indian religion founded in reaction to traditional Brahminical teachings, still practised today

Jnana yoga: the yoga of knowledge (of truth)

Karma: the idea that actions have consequences

Karma yoga: the yoga of action (in relation to status and one's role in life), and in relation to the non-attachment to the fruits of one's actions: *niskama* karma is action free from desire

Kleshwa: a mental defilement

Kundalini: latent female energy, believed to reside coiled at the base of the spine

Maharaja: a ruler of one of the principal native states of India

Mala: an illusion, which prevents us from seeing clearly our true nature

Mantra: a word or sound repeated in meditation to aid concentration or to imprint the sound of an element in the practitioner

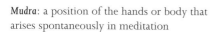

Mudra: a position of the hands or body that arises spontaneously in meditation

Nadi: a channel in the body through which *prana* flows

Niyama: observance

Non-dualism: the worldview that there is only one thing that exists in reality, e.g. consciousness

Prakrti: the principle of materiality; matter

Prana: the non-material body, made up of energy, not matter (or "food"), arising in the self and needed to support the individual

Pranayama: breath control

Pratyahara: redirecting the senses to the inner world

Purusha: the principle of pure consciousness, spirit, energy

Raja yoga: the royal yoga, usually taken to mean meditation

Samadhi: meditative consciousness

Samkhya: an influential school of Indian philosophy, closely related to yoga

Samskara: energetic knot in the body where conditioning and beliefs have got stuck

Satya: truthfulness

Shaivism: a religion/spiritual tradition based on the deity of Shiva; Kashmir Shaivism is a form of this tradition that was prevalent in the region of Kashmir, northern India

Shakti: a female deity conceptualized as the moving energy that makes up the entire manifest universe; as such, one half of the divine reality/consciousness, with Shiva as the other side

Shiva: a male deity conceptualized as pure consciousness, the transcendent; as such, one half of the divine reality/consciousness, with Shakti on the other side

Siddhi: power, both supernatural and worldly

Sramana: a striver; a renunciant man who practised yogic techniques to explore ideas of liberation

Sthira: ease of effort, especially in meditation

Sukha: steadiness of effort, especially in meditation

Sutra: a concise statement

Tantra: a theory, doctrine or books said to be divinely revealed; the system of practice and philosophical view of reality specified by these books

Tapas: the heat or fire generated by the discipline, devotion and hard work of the ascetic, which is needed to achieve liberation

Tarka: discernment

Tattva: a level of reality in the manifest world

Vairagya: dispassion

Vaishnavism: a religion/spiritual tradition based on the deity of Vishnu

Vedanta: a philosophy/spiritual tradition reflecting ideas from the end of the Vedic period

Vedas: canonical texts of Hinduism; texts from the Vedic period, 1500–500 BCE

Vinyasa: a flowing form of postural yoga

Vrittis: mental and emotional fluctuation, churning

Yama: restraint

References

Articles

Birch, J, "Unpublished Manuscript Evidence for the practice of numerous asanas in the 17th and 18th centuries", in *Yoga in Transformation: Historical and Contemporary Perspectives* edited by Karl Baier, Philipp A Maas and Karin Preisendanz (Vienna: V&R Unipress, 2018)

De Michelis, E, "Modern Yoga, History and Forms", in *Yoga in the Modern World: Contemporary Perspectives*, edited by Mark Singleton and Jean Byrne (London: Routledge, 2008)

Newcombe, S, "The Development of Modern Yoga: A Survey of the Field", *Religion Compass*, 25 November 2009

Singleton, M, "Yoga and Physical Culture: Transnational history and blurred discursive contexts", in *Routledge Handbook of Contemporary India*, edited by Knut A Jacobsen (London: Routledge, 2016)

Books

Bondy, D, *Yoga for Everyone: 50 poses for every type of body* (London: Dorling Kindersley, 2019)

Broad, W J, *The Science of Yoga: The risks and the rewards* (New York: Simon & Schuster, 2012)

Clark, B, *The Complete Guide to Yin Yoga: The Philosophy and Practice of Yin Yoga* (Canada: Wild Strawberry Productions, 2012)

Connolly, Peter, *A Student's Guide to the History and Philosophy of Yoga* (Sheffield: Equinox Publishing, 2014)

Cope, S, *Yoga and the Quest for True Self* (New York: Bantam Books, 2000)
— *The Great Work of Your Life* (New York: Bantam Books, 2012)

Farhi, D, *The Breathing Book* (London: St Martin's Griffin, 1996)
— *Bringing Yoga to Life* (London: HarperCollins, 2005)

Filmer Lorch, A, *Inside Meditation: In search of the unchanging nature within* (Leicester: Matador, 2012)

Jarmey, C, *The Concise Book of Muscles* (Chichester: Lotus Publishing, 2008)

Kaminoff, L and Matthews, A, *Yoga Anatomy: Your illustrated guide to postures, movements and breathing techniques* (Leeds: Human Kinetics, 2012)

Katie, B, *Loving What Is: Four questions that can change your life* (London: Rider, Ebury Publishing, 2002)

Kempton, S, *Awakening Shakti* (Louisville, CO: Sounds True Inc., 2013)

Lasater, J H, *Living Your Yoga: Finding the spiritual in everyday life* (Boulder, CO: Rodmell Press, 2015)
— *Restore and Rebalance: Yoga for deep relaxation* (Boulder, CO: Shambala Publishing, 2017)

Lesondak, D, *Fascia: What it is and why it matters* (Pencaitland: Handspring Publishing, 2017)

Mallinson, J and Singleton, M, *Roots of Yoga* (London: Penguin Classics, 2017)

Myers, T, *Anatomy Trains: Myofascial Meridians for Manual and Movement Therapists* (London: Churchill Livingstone, 2013)

Neill, G, *5 Common Yoga Injuries and How to Avoid Them* (Shut Up & Yoga blog e-book, 2019)

Roach, M G, *How Yoga Works* (Wayne, NJ: Diamond Cutter Press, 2004)

Samuel, G, *The Origins of Yoga and Tantra* (Cambridge: Cambridge University Press, 2008)

Saraswati, N, *Prana and Pranayama* (Bihar, India: Yoga Publications Trust, 2009)

Satyananda, S, *Asana, Pranayama, Mudra and Bandha* (Bihar, India: Yoga Publications Trust, 2003)

Singleton, M, *The Yoga Body: The origins of modern posture practice* (Oxford: Oxford University Press, 2010)

Stirk, J, *The Original Body: Primal movement for yoga teachers* (Pencaitland: Handspring Publishing, 2015)

Swanson, A, *The Science of Yoga: Understand the anatomy and physiology to perfect your practice* (London: Dorling Kindersley, 2019)

Wallis, C, *Tantra Illuminated: The philosophy, history and practices of a timeless tradition* (Pettaluma, CA: Mattamayura Press, 2013)

—— *The Recognition Sutras: Illuminating a 1000 year old masterpiece* (Pettaluma, CA: Mattamayura Press, 2017)

Wildcroft, T, *Post-lineage Yoga: From Guru to #MeToo* (Sheffield: Equinox Publishing, 2020)

Social Media/Online

Brea Johnson: www.heartandbonesyoga.com/

Julie Martin: www.brahmaniyoga.com/

Dr Garrett Neill: shutupandyoga.com/

Jesal Parikh and Tejal Petal: www.yogaisdeadpodcast.com

Matthew Remski: www.matthewremski.com

Laurent Roure: www.yogalaurent.com

Kathryn Bruni Young: kathrynbruniyoung.com/

Other

Gary Carter anatomy course: www.naturalbodies.co.uk/

School of Oriental and African Studies (SOAS) Centre of Yoga Studies at the University of London: www.soas.ac.uk/yoga-studies/

Yogacampus history of yoga course: www.yogacampus.com/online/a-history-of-yoga-the-latest-research

Index

Acknowledgements

I wouldn't be where I am today without the support of my teachers and students, especially Julie Martin. Thanks to my editor, Clare Churly, and designer, Yasia Williams, for their patience and encouragement; thanks also to Stephanie Jackson for approaching me after class one day about writing a yoga book. Finally, much love and thanks to my family and friends.

About the Author

Lucy Lucas is a mindfulness and yoga teacher who began her practice after spending a career in finance and consultancy. She trained in Bali, first taught yoga in Ibiza and now has a practice based in the UK, where she teaches classes and leads retreats.

www.lucylucas.com
🐦 @lucylucasyoga
📷 @lucylucasyoga

Also Available

Godsfield Companion: Chakras
Godsfield Companion: Crystals
Godsfield Companion: Mindfulness